THE WAR ON CANCER

The War on Cancer

An Anatomy of Failure, A Blueprint for the Future

by

GUY B. FAGUET

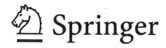 Springer

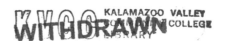

A C.I.P. Catalogue record for this book is available from the Library of Congress.

ISBN-10   1-4020-3618-3 (HB)
ISBN-10   1-4020-3617-5 (e-book)
ISBN-13   978-1-4020-3618-7 (HB)
ISBN-13   978-1-4020-3617-0 (e-book)

Published by Springer,
P.O. Box 17, 3300 AA Dordrecht, The Netherlands.

www.springeronline.com

Printed on acid-free paper

Cover figure:
The Anatomy Lesson of Dr. Nicolaes Tulp by Rembrandt
© (2005) Photo Scala, Florence

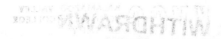

ABOUT THE AUTHOR

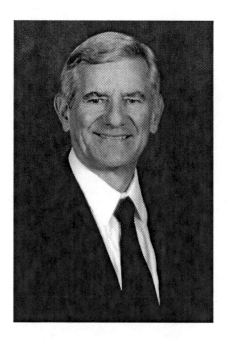

After receiving his MD degree from the Pontificia Universidad Javeriana in Bogota, Colombia, Dr. Faguet pursued postgraduate studies in Internal Medicine at the University of Texas Medical Branch and in Hematology/Oncology at Ohio State University, leading to an academic career at the Medical College of Georgia. His clinical and "bench" research, much of it in cell biology and leukemia, was funded by the National Institutes of Health and the Department of Veterans Affairs for 28 years, leading to the publication of 140 peer-reviewed articles, 7 book chapters, and two previous books on cancer. Dr. Faguet was a member of numerous medical societies and an ad hoc reviewer for the National Cancer Institute, the National Science Foundation and the Department of Veterans Affairs and for a number of prestigious medical journals. Since retiring, he devotes more time to his hobbies: classical music, jogging, portraiture, and traveling.

ACKNOWLEDGEMENTS

To Maria Teresa, Jean Paul, and Michèle

I am indebted to Dr. Jean-Paul G. Faguet, for invaluable advice on the organization and content of this book, to Dr. John C. Bailar for insightful comments and suggestions, and to Drs. Harvey Schipper, Gerald E. Marti, and Neil Caporaso for useful observations. All remaining errors are my own.

"Ce qui est vraiment extraordinaire, dans cette affaire, c'est le nombre et la qualité des "égarés". Il ne s'agit pas de demi-savants, d'extravagants, d'amis du merveilleux ; non, ce sont de vrais hommes de science, désintéressés, probes, habitués aux méthodes et aux mesures de laboratoire, des hommes à la tête froide et solide, et qui, soit avant soit après l'aventure, ont fait leurs preuves de chercheurs."

What is surprising, in this affair, is the numbers and qualifications of those gone astray. They were not half-wits, fools, or friends of the wondrous; No, they were true men of science, unbiased and honest men familiar with the scientific method: Men with cool and solid heads who, before and after their escapade, proved themselves worthy researchers.

Jean Rostand, *Confidences d'un biologiste*, Presses Pocket, Paris, 1990

TABLE OF CONTENTS

PREFACE

This book examines the root causes of three decades of disappointing progress in cancer treatment despite vast human and financial resources allocated towards its conquest since enactment of the National Cancer Act of 1971 and the extraordinary advances in molecular genetics of the last 20 years. It also identifies broad-based and far-reaching changes necessary to refocus drug development and clinical cancer research, and redirect cancer management. Opinions and proposals offered in this book emerged from the author's 30-year experience as a researcher and clinician that witnessed the widening disconnect between momentous advances in cancer research and the stagnation of cancer care delivery, and are supported by current medical literature.

Researchers and clinicians of my generation began their career at an auspicious time. Advances in histopathologic classifications[1], new procedures to diagnose and stage cancer[2-4], and the advent of powerful radiotherapy-delivery systems and administration schemes along with new cancer drugs marked the dawn of an era when the conquest of cancer seemed an attainable goal. Growing interest in cancer led to the recognition of Medical, Surgical, and Radiation Oncology as distinct specialty fields. It also fostered the emergence of multi-institutional cancer study groups dedicated to optimizing cancer management through the objective assessment of outcomes of patients treated under strict protocol guidelines. These cumulative advances led to early triumphs such as the near conquest of Hodgkin's disease, spearheaded by Kaplan[5] and DeVita[6], a century and a half after its description by Thomas Hodgkin[7]. However, this momentous event was to remain nearly isolated. Indeed, little additional progress has been made towards the cure of most invasive cancers. In fact, in the last 20 years, only testicular cancer has been added to the short list of malignancies routinely curable using chemotherapy [8].

Analysis of cancer incidence and death rates in the United States since 1930 reveals two opposing trends. Ominously, there was a sharp and continuous rise in lung cancer incidence and mortality in men that peaked in 1991-1992. This was followed by a comparable rise in women's that trails men's by 30 years, paralleling the smoking habits of both sexes. Alternatively, over the same period we witnessed a significant and progressive decline in death rates for stomach cancer in both sexes, for uterine and colon-rectal cancers in women, and more recently lung cancer in men. However, these declines are largely attributable to prevention and early-stage detection, to food refrigeration, to improved infection control and transfusion therapy, to enhanced nursing, social, and rehabilitation services, and to better general medical support, rather than to advances in cancer treatment. This is because the vast human and financial resources, unleashed by the National Cancer Act of 1971, were undermined by flawed hypotheses regarding the nature of cancer and by reliance on trial and error or serendipity as the main forces driving anti-cancer drug development. As a result, disease eradication is currently achievable in only 11 of over 200 human malignancies and meaningful survival prolongation is possible for another few [9,10]. These are meager achievements considering that the first remissions in acute leukemia was reported in 1948 [11], and the first cure of a disseminated solid tumor (choriocarcinoma) was achieved five years later. In the interim, the enormous progress in understanding cancer biology, genetics, and growth regulation made over the last 20 years has only recently began to spawn clinical applications. To quote the President's Cancer Panel 1999 report, albeit in a different context, "*if we do not bridge the persistent disconnect between the research and delivery enterprises, our progress against suffering and mortality from cancer will continue to be slow, uneven, and incremental*" [12].

Hence, my analysis of the numerous and complex issues responsible for the stagnation in cancer therapies of the last 30 years was designed to foster a critical awareness of the forces that perpetuate the *War on Cancer* policies of the past and to propose a way forward. Issues examined include the impacting role of clinicians, clinical researchers, their sponsors and publishers, and of the mass media, and the clinical, research, and drug development consequences of viewing cancer as a new growth to be eradicated at all cost, rather than as a genetic cellular dysfunction that can be prevented, detected early, and controlled genetically. I acknowledge that implementation of this three-prong cancer control proposal requires the enlightened cooperation and participation of health-care professionals, policy-makers, and of the public at large. However, the imperatives of reversing current cancer incidence and mortality trends, a goal not achievable under the current cancer cell-kill paradigm, and of reducing the 1,500 daily deaths from cancer in the United States and tens of thousands more around the world, provide powerful incentives for an overdue change in direction.

REFERENCES:

1. Lukes RJ, Carver LF, Hall TC, Rappaport H & Rubin T. Report of the nomenclature committee. Cancer Res 26:1311,1966.
2. Rosenberg SA. Report of the committee on the staging of Hodgkin's disease. Cancer Res 26:1310,1966.
3. Hreschchyshyn M, Sheehan FR & Holland JF. Visualization of retroperitoneal lymph nodes. Lymphangiography as an aid in the measurement of tumor growth. Cancer 14:205-209,1961.
4. Enright LP, Trueblood HW & Nelsen TS. The surgical diagnosis of abdominal Hodgkin's disease. Surg Gynec Obst 130:853-858,1970.
5. Hodgkin T. On some morbid appearances of the absorbent glands and spleen. Medico-Chirurgical Transactions 17:68-114,1832.
6. Rosenberg SA, Kaplan H, Hoppe RT, et al. The Stanford randomized trials of the treatment of Hodgkin's disease: 1967-1980. In Rosenberg HS and Kaplan H, eds. Malignant lymphomas: etiology, immunology, pathology, treatment. Bristol-Myers cancer symposia. Vol 3. New York: Academic Press, 1982.
7. DeVita VT, Jr, Simon RM, Hubbard SM, et al. Curability of advanced Hodgkin's disease with chemotherapy: long-term follow-up of MOPP-treated patients at the National Cancer Institute (NCI). Ann Intern Med 92:587-595,1980.
8. Einhorn LH and Stephens DW. Chemotherapy of disseminated testicular cancer: a random prospective study. Cancer 46:1339-1344,1980.
9. Krakoff IH. Systemic treatment of cancer. CA-A Cancer J Clin 46:136-141,1996.
10. Holland JF, Frei E, Kuffe DW, Bast RC. Principles of medical oncology. Cancer Medicine e.5 Online http://www.cancer.org/eprise/main/docroot/PUB/content/PUB_2_1_Cancer_Medicine_e5Online?
11. Farber S, Diamond LK, Mercer RD, Sylvester RF, Wolff JA. Temporary remissions in acute leukemia in children produced by folic acid antagonist, 4-aminopteroylglutamic acid (Aminopterin). New Engl J Med 238:787-793,1948.
12. The National Cancer Program: Assessing the past, charting the future, 1999 Annual Report. http:\\deainfo.nci.nih.gov/ADVISORY/pcp/pcp99rpt/99report.htm

INTRODUCTION

The message of this book is that, contrary to recurrent announcements of breakthroughs in the *War on Cancer* designed to influence policy makers and impress the public, little progress has been made in the treatment of cancer since the enactment of the *National Cancer Act of 1971*. Thus, the purpose of this book is two-fold. The first is to identify the reasons why vast human and financial resources devoted in the last thirty years to the conquest of cancer, the stated goal of the *National Cancer Act of 1971*, have failed to do so. The second is to propose cogent, evidence-driven cancer control measures needed to succeed. In order to dissect a highly complex subject, I will present an orderly analysis of the multifaceted aspects of cancer focusing primarily on Medical Oncology, the specialty entrusted with the treatment of disseminated cancer with systemic chemotherapy. First, the enormous impact of cancer on the nation will be highlighted by a brief analysis of its cost in human and financial terms, and by a review of its incidence and mortality statistics. Our inability to significantly impact either will be demonstrated by the dismal cure and survival rates achieved today, and by unchanging trends. The evolution through the ages of speculative ideas about the nature of cancer will be briefly outlined for historical perspective and as a prelude to reviewing theories and hypotheses of the last thirty years about its origin and treatment. The inevitable impact of these theories and hypotheses on drug development and patient care will be contrasted to the vast body of scientific data revealing the true nature of cancer, thus highlighting the growing dichotomy between cancer research at the laboratory level and cancer management in the clinical setting. Then, I will identify crucial influences exerted by a cohort of interested parties that, whether directly or indirectly involved with cancer management, have fostered and help preserve the gap between bench research and patient care.

These include the formidable influence of the National Cancer Institute that steers cancer research and patient care through selective allocation of funds, the growing presence and impact of profit-driven pharmaceutical companies, the role of professional publications in shaping Oncologists' attitudes and practices, and of the mass media in molding patients' perceptions and expectations. Our virtual journey will take us to the inescapable conclusion that the cell-kill approach to cancer management, an enduring legacy of the germ origin of cancer and other past misconceptions discredited by recent advances in cancer genetics, has failed to achieve its objectives. This, in turn, will lead me to propose new cancer control strategies. These strategies, grounded in the knowledge that cancer cells, unlike pathogenic bacteria, are genetically altered self-cells and not foreign invaders that must be exterminated at all cost, call for a sequential approach to cancer control. This includes prevention and early detection, and when these fail, molecularly targeted therapies designed to prevent, revert, or control the aberrant genetic pathways responsible for the development, growth, and dissemination of cancer, rather than to the extermination of the cells that harbor them. The new paradigm calls upon medical researchers to develop simple, specific, and cost-effective screening tools for the early detection of all cancers, and to exploit the vast genomic database towards translational therapies for patients with advanced or progressive malignancies. It also calls upon policy makers to enact enlightened public policies designed to develop and implement cancer prevention and screening programs of national scope and achievable goals, and to redirect clinical research funding towards evidence-based projects focused on patient- rather than tumor-outcomes.

The sources of much of the scientific evidence cited in this book, as revealed by the list of references, originate in the United States. However, cancer incidence and mortality are influenced more by factors that are common to all people than by ethnicity or geography, by a failure of all nations to implement cancer prevention policies, by the inadequacy of current screening procedures, and by the inefficacy of drugs available today to treat advanced cancer. Given these circumstances, which tend to equalize cancer incidence rates and treatment outcomes in rich and poor countries, our conclusions and our proposals are applicable beyond our borders.

PART I

CANCER STATISTICS: SOME FACTS

Chapter 1

ASSESSING THE MAGNITUDE OF THE PROBLEM

The cost of cancer in the United States, in terms of human suffering and financial resources, is enormous. Since 1990, over 6 million Americans have died of cancer, more than the combined casualties from the Civil war, WWII, and the Vietnam and Korea conflicts combined. Over their lifetime, about 1 out of 2 American men and 1 out of 3 American women will develop cancer [1]. The National Institutes of Health estimate overall costs for cancer in the United Sates in the year 2002 at approximately $171.6 billion, including $60.9 billion for direct medical costs, $15.5 billion for indirect costs of morbidity (lost productivity due to illness), and $95.2 billion for indirect mortality costs (lost productivity due to premature death) [2]. In 1997, the last year for which data are available, 5 billion dollars were allocated to laboratory cancer research in the United States[3]. Yet, despite extraordinary advances in our understanding the biology, genetics, and growth regulation of cancer, little progress has been made towards its prevention and treatment. Indeed, in 2004 over 1.3 million Americans will develop cancer and more than 560.000 will die of it [4] (Table I). Because cancer deaths shorten the average life-span by 15.1 years per person, an estimated total of 8.3 million years of life were lost from cancer deaths in 1998. This exceeds the years of life lost from heart disease deaths (7.8 million years), and from all other causes of death combined (6.5 million years) [5]. Finally, because the vast majority of cancers afflict individuals 55 years of age or older it was estimated, based on population projections from the US Bureau of the Census [6], that 1 in 56 Americans in this age group contracted cancer during 2001 and 1 in 130 died of the disease.

1.   CANCER STATISTICS

1.1   How are statistics collected?

In the United States, the Surveillance, Epidemiology and End Results (SEER) Program of the National Cancer Institute (NCI) began collecting cancer incidence and survival data on January 1, 1973 from the states of Connecticut, Iowa, New Mexico, Utah, and Hawaii and the metropolitan areas of Detroit and San Francisco-Oakland. In 1974-1975, Atlanta and the 13 Seattle-Puget Sound counties were added, as were 10 predominantly black rural counties in Georgia (1978) and American Indian areas in Arizona (1980). In 1992 minority Hispanic populations living in Los Angeles county and the San Jose-Monterrey area were added. In 2001, coverage was expanded to Kentucky, New Jersey, and the previously uncovered portions of California. Information on cancer cases is also collected by NCI from Alaska natives. Thus, SEER overall coverage reaches approximately 65 million persons or 26% of the US population, compared to 35 million previously [1]. Although SEER does not cover the entire US population, validation studies with the recorded cause of death for 17 cancer sites representing two thirds of cancer cases in the United States revealed a 90% correlation [7].

Cancer mortality data are collected by the National Center for Health Statistics, through mandated death certificates completed by physicians and coroners. Both are published annually in the SEER Cancer Statistics Review, and are also available in the web at www-seer.ims.nci.nih.org. Since 1997 the Centers for Disease Control and Prevention supports cancer registries in 45 states, 3 territories, and the District of Columbia: 45 for enhancing established registries and 4 for developing and implementing new registries [8]. Cancer incidence and mortality data are available through the North American Association of Central Cancer Registries, directly and through their web site: www.naaccr.org. In addition to these population-based registries, hospital tumor boards maintain cancer incidence and mortality data for their particular facility. However, in contrast to population-based surveillance data that reflect national rates and trends, hospital registries reflect the type of practice, catchment area, and other factors peculiar to each institution.

At the international level, cancer data are compiled by the International Agency for Research on Cancer (IARC), an arm of the World Health Organization (WHO). Because few countries maintain nationwide cancer surveillance programs, relying instead on regional databases, IARC uses mortality data reported to the WHO by each country to estimate cancer incidence. Thus, the validity of cancer data is influenced by the country of origin, the accuracy of death certificates, and by many other factors.

1.2   How statistics are reported and what they mean [9]

Both cancer incidence and mortality can be expressed as total number of cases for a specific population over a particular time period. For example, more than 1.3 million new cancer cases are anticipated in the United States in 2004 [4]. However, total cancer cases vary with population size and age composition, thus precluding comparing cancer incidence trends over time in the same country, or among countries with populations of different size and age distribution. This problem can be solved by expressing the number of cancer cases per 100,000 people in the total population, or in any segment thereof (males, whites, etc), adjusted for age makeup. The latter is necessary because cancer is a disease that predominates in the elderly. For example, in the US over 75% of invasive cancers occur in the 20% of Americans 55 years of age or older [10]. Hence, the incidence of prostate cancer in 1997 can be reported as 64.1 per 100,000 total population (male and female), as 147.0 per 100,000 men, or further broken down by age groups. These adjustments enable comparing cancer rates over time in the same country and among countries with different population size and age composition. There is, however, one caveat: in the United States age adjustment is based on the 1970 United States census (recently re-adjusted to the 2000 population census), whereas most international age-adjusted data reported by the IARC are standardized to a 1960 world standard population. Thus, caution must be exercised when comparing cancer data from different countries when they are adjusted to the same standard population. Unless otherwise specified, all references to cancer incidence and mortality rates in this book will be population- and age-adjusted.

1.3   Cancer incidence and mortality in the United States, 2004

The American Cancer Society publishes yearly estimates of the numbers of new cancer cases and cancer deaths expected in the United States, based on last available actual rates (usually 5 years in arrears) projected onto yearly estimates of the size and age distribution of the United States population. While these estimates are only projections they have proved reasonably accurate when compared to actual data gathered and tabulated several years later, thus justifying their interim use. The American Cancer Society estimates that 1,368,030 Americans will develop cancer in 2004: 699,560 men and 668,470 women 4 (Table I). While there are over 200 different types of cancer, their relative incidence is highly uneven. Indeed, approximately 2/3 of all male and female cancers predicted for 2004 are accounted for by five cancers (Figure 1). According to the same source, 563,700 Americans will die of cancer in 2004: 290,890 men and 272,810 women [4] (Table I). Five cancers will account for approximately 62% of all cancer deaths in American men and women (Figure 1) in 2004. These same cancers accounted for a similar fraction of all cancer deaths in American men and women recorded in 1995 [11] (Table II).

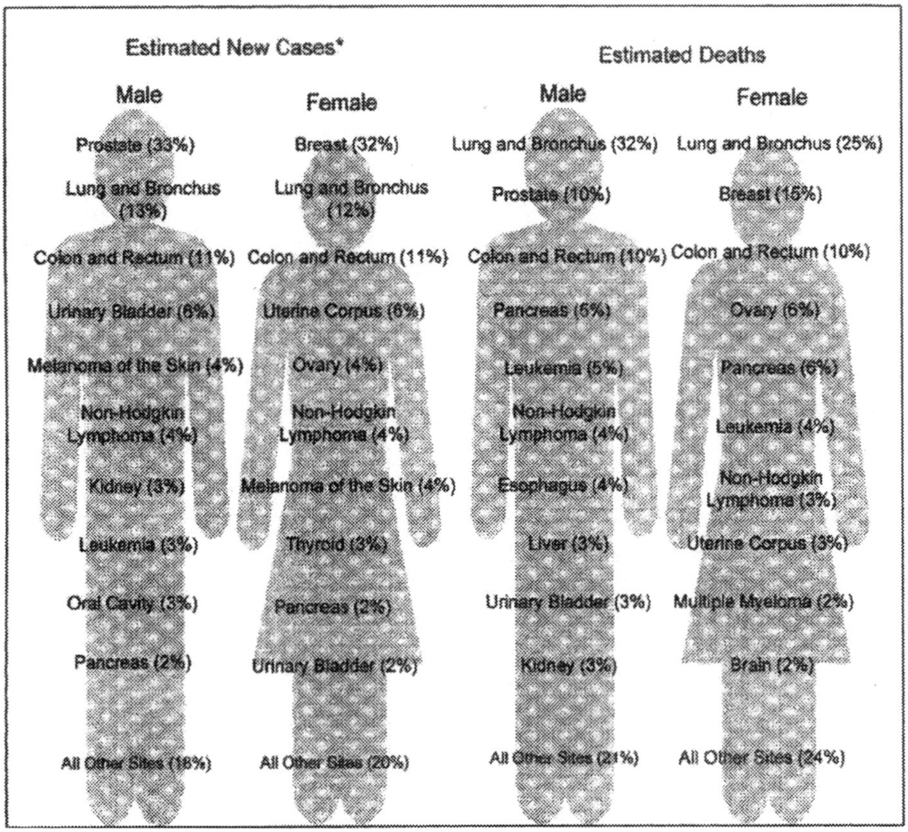

Figure 1. Ten leading cancers (as percent of new cases and deaths), by sex: US estimates 2004 (Reproduced with permission from Cancer Statistics, 2004, CA Cancer J Clin 54: 8-29,2004, (ref #4)

Table I. Estimated new cancer cases and cancer deaths by sex for all sites: US 2004 (Reproduced with permission from CA Cancer J Clin 2004 54: 8-29, 2004 (ref 4).

	Estimated New Cases			Estimated Deaths		
	Both Sexes	Male	Female	Both sexes	Male	Female
All Sites	1,368,030	699,560	668,470	563,700	290,890	272,810
Oral cavity & pharynx	28,260	18,550	9,710	7,230	4,830	2,400
Tongue	7,320	4,860	2,460	1,700	1,100	600
Mouth	10,080	5,410	4,670	1,890	1,070	820
Pharynx	8,250	6,330	1,920	2,070	1,460	610
Other oral cavity	2,610	1,950	660	1,570	1,200	370
Digestive system	255,640	135,410	120,230	134,840	73,240	61,600
Esophagus	14,250	10,860	3,390	13,300	10,250	3,050
Stomach	22,710	13,640	9,070	11,780	6,900	4,880
Small intestine	5,260	2,750	2,510	1,130	610	520
Colon†	106,370	50,400	55,970	56,730	28,320	28,410
Rectum	40,570	23,220	17,350			
Anus, anal canal, & anorectum	4,010	1,890	2,120	580	210	370
Liver & intrahepatic bile duct	18,920	12,580	6,340	14,270	9,450	4,820
Gallbladder & other biliary	6,950	2,960	3,990	3,540	1,290	2,250
Pancreas	31,860	15,740	16,120	31,270	15,440	15,830
Other digestive organs	4,740	1,370	3,370	2,240	770	1,470
Respiratory system	186,550	102,730	83,820	165,130	95,460	69,670
Larynx	10,270	8,060	2,210	3,830	3,010	820
Lung & bronchus	173,770	93,110	80,660	160,440	91,930	68,510
Other respiratory organs	2,510	1,560	950	860	520	340
Bones & joints	2,440	1,230	1,210	1,300	720	580
Soft tissue (including heart)	8,680	4,760	3,920	3,660	2,020	1,640
Skin (excluding basal & squamous)	59,350	31,640	27,710	10,250	6,590	3,660
Melanoma-skin	55,100	29,900	25,200	7,910	5,050	2,860
Other nonepithelial skin	4,910	2,400	2,510	2,340	1,540	800
Breast	217,440	1,450	215,990	40,580	470	40,110
Genital system	323,210	240,660	82,550	59,250	30,530	28,720
Uterine cervix	10,520		10,520	3,900		3,900
Uterine corpus	40,320		40,320	7,090		7,090
Ovary	25,580		25,580	16,090		16,090
Vulva	3,970		3,970	850		850
Vagina & other genital, female	2,160		2,160	790		790
Prostate	230,110	230,110		29,900	29,900	
Testis	8,980	8,980		360	360	
Penis & other genital, male	1,570	1,570		270	270	
Urinary system	98,400	68,290	30,110	25,880	17,060	8,820
Urinary bladder	60,240	44,640	15,600	12,710	8,780	3,930
Kidney & renal pelvis	35,710	22,080	13,630	12,480	7,870	4,610
Ureter & other urinary organs	2,450	1,570	880	690	410	280
Eye & orbit	2,090	1,130	960	180	110	70
Brain & other nervous system	18,400	10,540	7,860	12,690	7,200	5,490
Endocrine system	25,520	6,950	18,570	2,440	1,140	1,300
Thyroid	23,600	5,960	17,640	1,460	620	840
Other endocrine	1,920	990	930	980	520	460
Lymphoma	62,250	33,180	29,070	20,730	11,090	9,640
Hodgkin disease	7,880	4,330	3,550	1,320	700	620
Non-Hodgkin lymphoma	54,370	28,850	25,520	19,410	10,390	9,020
Multiple myeloma	15,270	8,090	7,180	11,070	5,430	5,640
Leukemia	33,440	19,020	14,420	23,300	12,990	10,310
Acute lymphocytic leukemia	3,830	2,110	1,720	1,450	820	630
Chronic lymphocytic leukemia	8,190	5,050	3,140	4,800	2,730	2,070
Acute myeloid leukemia	11,920	6,280	5,640	8,870	4,810	4,060
Chronic myeloid leukemia	4,600	2,700	1,900	1,570	940	630
Other leukemia‡	4,900	2,880	2,020	6,610	3,690	2,920
Other & unspecified primary sites‡	31,090	15,930	15,160	45,170	22,010	23,160

Table II. Cancer mortality: projections for 2004 vs reported for 1995. From CA Cancer J Clin 54:8-29,2004 (ref #4), and Cancer Medicine[e], 2000 (ref #12).

	Predicted for 2004		Reported for 1995	
	Number of cases	*Percentage*	*Number of cases*	*Percentage*
Men				
All sites	290,890	100.0	281,611	100.0
Lung-Bronchus	91,930	31.6	91,800	32.6
Prostate	29,900	10.3	34,475	12.2
Colorectal	28,320	9.7	28,409	10.0
Pancreas	15.440	5.3	12,826	4.6
Non-Hodgkin's	10,390	3.6	11,597	4.1
Women				
All sites	272,810	100.0	256,644	100.0
Lung-Bronchus	68,510	25.1	59,304	23.0
Breast	40,110	14.7	43,844	17.0
Colorectal	28,410	10.4	29,237	11.4
Pancreas	15,830	5.8	13,940	5.4
Ovary	16,090	5.9	13,342	5.2

1.4   Individual probability of developing [4] and dying [12] of cancer in the US

Based on 1998-2000 data, the cumulative life-long risk of developing cancer was almost 1 in 2 for an American male and more than 1 in 3 for an American female (Table IIIa). Likewise, the cumulative life-long risk of dying from cancer was nearly 1 in 4 for an American male and 1 in 5 for an American female (Table IIIb). However, the risk of developing and dying of cancer and the type of cancer involved are gender- and age-dependent. For example, while the male cumulative life-long risk of dying from prostate cancer (1 in 28) is virtually identical to a woman's cumulative risk of dying of breast cancer (1 in 29), only 1 in nearly 13,000 men will develop prostate cancer before age 40, whereas only 1 woman in 229 will develop breast cancer by the same age (Table IIIb). In 1999, the leading cause of cancer death in men ages 20 to 39 was leukemia, whereas it was lung cancer after age 40. In contrast, in women the risk of developing leukemia was highest before age 20, whereas breast cancer prevailed between ages 20 and 60, and lung cancer predominated after age 60. However, as increasing numbers of smoking adolescent females come to age, mortality rates from lung cancer will shift to younger age groups, eventually replacing breast cancer after age 40.

Table - III. Percentage (and odds) probability of developing (IIIA) or dying (IIIB) from one of the four most common invasive cancers, by sex. Reproduced with permission from Cancer Medicine, 2000 (ref #12).

III A		Birth to 39	40 to 59	60 to 79	Birth to Death
All sites	Men	1.36 (1 in 73)	8.0 (1 in 12)	33.9 (1 in 3)	44.8 (1 in 2)
	Women	1.92 (1 in 52)	9.0 (1 in 11)	22.6 (1 in 4)	38.0 (1 in 3)
Breast	Women	0.44 (1 in 229)	4.1 (1 in 24)	7.5 (1 in 13)	13.4 (1 in 78)
Colon	Men	0.06 (1 in 1,678)	0.9 (1 in 116)	3.9 (1 in 25)	5.9 (1 in 17)
	Women	0.06 (1 in 1,651)	0.7 (1 in 150)	3.1 (1 in 33)	5.5 (1 in 18)
Lung	Men	0.03 (1 in 3,439)	1.0 (1 in 98)	5.8 (1 in 17)	7.7 (1 in 13)
	Women	0.03 (1 in 3,046)	0.8 (1 in 126)	3.9 (1 in 25)	5.7 (1 in 17)
Prostate	Men	0.01 (1 in 12,833)	2.3 (1 in 44)	14.2 (1 in 7)	17.2 (1 in 6)

III B		Birth to 39	40 to 59	60 to 79	Birth to Death
All sites	Men	0.31 (1 in 325)	2.9 (1 in 34)	15.3 (1 in 7)	23.5 (1 in 4)
	Women	0.31 (1 in 319)	2.9 (1 in 35)	11.3 (1 in 9)	20.5 (1 in 5)
Breast	Women	0.07 (1 in 1,436)	0.8 (1 in 131)	1.8 (1 in 57)	3.4 (1 in 29)
Colon	Men	0.02 (1 in 5,129)	0.3 (1 in 358)	1.6 (1 in 64)	2.5 (1 in 41)
	Women	0.02 (1 in 6,655)	0.2 (1 in 485)	1.1 (1 in 88)	2.5 (1 in 41)
Lung	Men	0.02 (1 in 5,173)	0.9 (1 in 107)	5.2 (1 in 19)	6.8 (1 in 15)
	Women	0.02 (1 in 5,930)	0.6 (1 in 156)	3.1 (1 in 32)	4.5 (1 in 22)
Prostate	Men	0.01 (1 in 10,000)	0.1 (1 in 1,312)	1.8 (1 in 56)	3.5 (1 in 28)

2. CANCER PREVALENCE IN THE US, 2000

Cancer prevalence refers to the number or proportion of individuals with any type of cancer, but for non-melanoma skin cancers, alive at any given time regardless of when the diagnosis was established and whether they are cured, dying of the disease, or somewhere in between. In essence, prevalence includes all cases of new and preexisting cancers that are alive at a particular time regardless of cancer status. Thus, collection of such data requires a sufficient period of time to capture all previously diagnosed cases. In the US, the Connecticut Registry is the only registry with sufficient follow-up data (cancers diagnosed after 1935) enabling calculation of cancer prevalence. Prevalence data from this regional registry is extrapolated nation-wide based on the US population. The major interest of cancer prevalence data is to policy-makers for it identifies the level of human and financial burden imposed by cancer on the health care system and the level of support required from public and private sources. As of January 2000, 9,555,312 Americans were alive with cancer: 4,241,699 (44%) of these were men and 5,313,613 (56%) were women [5]. The four most prevalent cancers accounted for 60% of all cancer patients alive in 2000 [13]. They were: female breast (22% of the total), prostate (17%), colorectal (11%), and gynecologic (10%) cancer. Men accounted for 100% of prostate and 73% of urinary bladder cancers. Women accounted for 100% of uterine and 99% of breast cancers. Survivors of colorectal cancer and melanoma of the skin were fairly evenly distributed between the genders.

3.   HISTORICAL TRENDS: INCIDENCE, MORTALITY AND SURVIVAL, 1950-2000

3.1   Incidence and mortality

In the United States, the total number of new cancer cases between 1950 and 2000 [4,12,14] rose by 1.5% annually from an age- and population-adjusted incidence rate of 248 to 476 (table IV). Likewise, total cancer deaths rose by 0.1% per year from an adjusted mortality rate of 194 to 200 [5].

Table - IV. Changes in cancer incidence and mortality, 1950-99 & 5-year survival rates Reproduced from SEER Cancer Statistics Review 1975-2000, ref #5. APC*, annual % change.

	All races, 2000		Whites			
	Cases	Deaths	% change, 1950-2000 in		5-year survival	
			Incidence	Mortality	Rates (%)	
			Total APC*	Total APC	1950-54	92-99
Oral	30,200	7,492	-31.2 -0.5	-49.7 -1.2	46	59.7
Esophagus	12,300	12,232	16.0 0.7	26.9 0.6	4	15.4
Stomach	21,500	12,645	-74.3 -2.2	-83.3 -3.5	12	21.4
Colon	93,800	48,570	40.7 0.4	-25.6 -0.5	41	63.0
Rectum	36,400	8,907	-12.8 -0.4	-68.6 -2.7	40	63.0
Liver	15,300	16,582	294.9 2.5	27.3 0.6	1	6.8
Pancreas	28,300	29,331	36.5 0.3	21.3 0.1	1	4.4
Larynx	10,100	3,861	43.0 0.2	-23.3 -0.5	52	66.6
Lung	164,100	155,788	294.3 2.3	270.0 2.3	6	15.1
Men	89,500	90,676	206.7 1.4	203.9 1.7	5	13.4
Women	74,600	65,112	697.4 4.4	611.5 4.4	9	17.2
Melanoma	47,700	7,420	619.1 4.3	165.1 1.8	49	89.8
Breast, women	182,800	41,872	90.6 1.5	-19.5 -0.2	60	87.9
Cervix	12,800	4,200	-77.6 -2.4	-79.1 -3.5	59	72.9
Uterus	36,100	6,585	18.5 -0.2	-68.6 -2.1	72	86.3
Ovary	23,100	14,453	15.7 0.4	3.6 -0.2	30	52.4
Prostate	180,400	31,078	282.9 3.3	-4.0 0.3	43	98.4
Testis	6,900	338	167.6 2.1	-72.6 -3.0	57	95.8
Bladder	53,200	12,306	96.9 1.2	-31.0 -0.9	53	82.6
Kidney	31,200	12,038	196.1 2.2	42.4 0.7	34	62.9
Brain	16,500	12,655	159.7 1.3	58.0 0.8	21	32.1
Thyroid	18,400	1,328	240.8 2.1	-44.8 -1.6	80	96.1
Hodgkin's	7,400	1,287	21.0 0.2	-75.2 -3.3	30	85.0
Non-Hodgkin's	54,900	22,553	252.0 3.0	152.5 1.8	33	57.2
Myeloma	13,600	10,697	291.6 1.9	254.4 1.9	6	30.9

	All races, 2000		Whites					
	Cases	Deaths	% change, 1950-2000 in				5-year survival rates (%)	
			Incidence		Mortality			
			Total	APC*	Total	APC	1950-54	92-99
Leukemia	30,800	21,339	31.5	0.4	9.6	-0.2	10	47.6
Childhood	8,600	1,526	62.4	0.8	-69.0	-2.8	20	78.7
All Sites	1,220,100	553,080	88.7	1.5	0.4	0.1	35	64.4

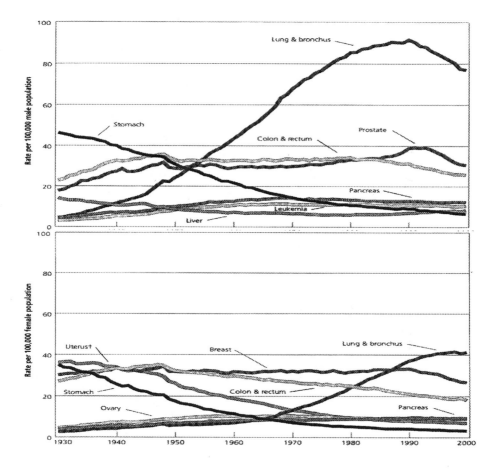

Figure -2. Age-adjusted cancer death rates in men (top) and women (bottom): 1930-2000 women. Reproduced with permission from, CA Cancer J Clin 54:8-29, 2004 (ref #4).

These changes were due mostly to the spectacular rise in lung cancer incidence which resulted in a near 4-fold increase in lung cancer mortality rates among men and a 6-fold upsurge among women, a rise not offset by a concomitant sharp fall in stomach, uterine, and other cancers with decreasing mortality rates (Figure 2). Gender differences in lung cancer incidence and mortality trends, and their relative timing parallel the gender-specific smoking habits, with women's smoking patterns trailing men's by approximately thirty years. Given the enormous impact of lung cancer on overall cancer statistics, statisticians and epidemiologists attempt to uncover underlying trends among other cancers by analyzing incidence and mortality data after excluding lung cancer. After excluding lung cancer, the overall cancer incidence between 1950 and 2000 rose 1.5% per year but mortality declined 0.4% per year [5] (Table IV). However, a detailed analysis of mortality trends is more sobering. Indeed, as shown in the figure, of the 28 most frequent cancers in the US, 10 experienced a yearly drop in mortality of 1% or greater but 6 saw their mortality increased by more than 1% a year. The latter accounted for 345,568 deaths in 2000 compared to 101,785 for the former [10], a ratio of over 3:1. Even after exclusion of lung cancer deaths in 2000 (155,788), the ratio remains nearly 2:1, which is to say that between 1950 and 2000 twice as many Americans died of cancers with increasing rather than with decreasing mortality rates. Furthermore, improvements in cancer mortality for 4 out 7 cancers declining by over 2% per year since 1950 (stomach cancer in both sexes, and in gynecologic and colorectal cancers in women) are attributable to the introduction of food refrigeration, to improved dietary and sanitary habits [15], to early detection [16], and to better supportive medical care, rather than to improved cancer therapy. The other 3 (childhood and germ cell malignancies) are chemotherapy-sensitive tumors that accounted for only 22,900 new cases and 3,146 deaths in 2000. More on this in chapter 7. There is however, good news: falling incidence (by 0.7% annually) between 1992 and 1995 and mortality rates (by 1% annually) between 1993 and 1998, with subsequent stabilization through 2000 (the latest available data) [10]. This potential trend, largely due to falling lung cancer incidence, is likely to continue if declining cigarette smoking observed among all races between 1965 and 2002 (Figure 3) continues. Likewise, behavioral changes in response to HIV infection are likely to reverse the rising incidence and mortality rates of non-Hodgkin's lymphoma observed since the mid-1980s. Such trend reversals underscore the powerful impact of behavioral changes on cancer prevention, and in turn the importance of including prevention in cancer control programs.

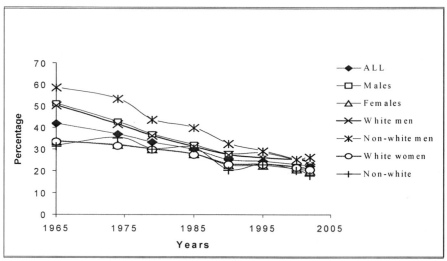

Figure -3. Trends in the prevalence of cigarette smoking among adult Americans: 1965-2002. (Source: National Center for Health Statistics. Health, United States 2004, with chartbook on Trends in the health of Americans. Hyattsville, MD. 2004).

3.2 Survival statistics

Aside from mortality rates, survival is also used to assess progress in cancer management, with 5-year relative survival (i.e. adjusted to survival of the same age-group in the general population) being favored. Comparisons of five-year survival rates reported by SEER for the 1950-54 and 1992-99 periods [5] suggest substantial survival gains for each cancer (Table IV). However, while these gains imply progress in the *War on Cancer*, their clinical relevance and their causes must be understood so that future plans can be drawn based on facts rather than perceptions. To address these issues, we will examine survival gains for the five most lethal cancers in the United States (Lung, Colorectal, Breast, Prostate, and Pancreas) that accounted for 57% of all cancer deaths in 2000 [12]. Five-year survival gains between 1950-54 and 1992-99 ranged from 1.5-fold for breast cancer to 4.4-fold for pancreatic cancer. However, a 4.4-fold improvement in 5-year survival in pancreatic cancer is meaningless as only approximately 4% of patients reached that landmark and the average survival for this cancer remains unchanged (3-4 months) since 1950. Likewise, lung cancer patients on the average live 7-9 months from diagnosis today despite a reported 2.5-fold improvement in 5-year survival since 1950-54. Moreover, while improvements in 5-year survival are frequently presented to the public and to policymakers as evidence of success in the *War on Cancer* they should not be. This is because while survival is a valid measure of treatment outcome within a clinical trial, it is misleading when applied over long periods of time [17]. Indeed, factors other than therapy affect survival favorably. They include improvements in supportive medical care and better screening and diagnostic tools. The latter two enable detection of more cases in curable and non-curable early stages of the disease. Because their cancer was diagnosed earlier in its course, these patients will survival longer (called *"lead-time bias"*) than individuals with more advanced disease diagnosed in the past [18] independently of their treatment.

An excellent example of the influence of early diagnosis on survival is documented for breast cancer in the SEER cancer statistics review, 1973-1997 [19], reproduced in Figure 4.

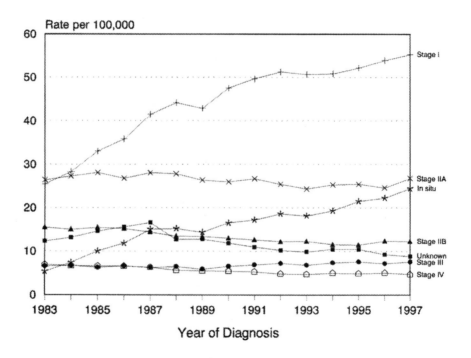

Figure -4. Female breast cancer incidence rates by stage, 1983-1997 (Reproduced from SEER Cancer Statistic Review, 1973-1997).

As shown, during this period the incidence of *in situ* and stage I breast cancer, the two earliest stages of this disease, increased 5- and 2-fold, respectively, as a consequence of the widespread adoption of mammography and public awareness. Not surprisingly, the incidence of the more advanced stages II, III and IV, detected by cruder methods such as CT or bone scans, or diagnosed when symptoms or tumor masses develop, began to decrease as more and more cases are detected at earlier stages. Because cancer mortality is directly proportional to disease stage, the more cases detected with early-stage disease the longer the survival of the overall group. The impact of early-stage detection on breast cancer incidence and mortality between 1973 and 1997 is supported by SEER statistics. Indeed, the sharp rise in the number of *in situ* and stage I breast cancer cases increased the overall breast cancer incidence by 0.4% per year, whereas their better prognosis reduced the overall breast cancer mortality by 2.1% per year. Similar trends were observed in prostate cancer after the widespread introduction of prostate-specific antigen (PSA) to screen for this disease in the late 1980s [16].

Chapter 2

THE PROBLEM IS GROWING, NOT GOING AWAY

In the U.S., the total number of cancer cases has increased year after year since cancer statistics have been kept. Indeed, while 12,769 Americans are reported to have died of cancer in 1900, representing 3.7% of total deaths (343,217), 158,335 cancer deaths were recorded in the US in 1940 and 553,768 in 2001, representing 11.2% and 23% of total deaths for those years (1,417,269 in 1940 and 2,416,425 in 2001) [20]. Although older statistics lack accuracy and precision, they serve to illustrate that while in 1900 cancer was the eighth cause of death in the US, it has risen to be second only to heart disease since 1940. This progressive rise is related to three major factors: a growing population, increasing longevity that places more individuals at risk of developing cancer, and disproportionate increases in cancer incidence rates associated with progressive age. Other contributing factors such as increased exposure to environmental carcinogens especially prevalent in industrialized societies and behavioral risks will be addressed in Chapter V, in the context of cancer prevention.

As reported by the US bureau of the Census [21] and plotted in Figure 5-top frame), the US population expanded by 86% between 1950 and 2000 (from 151.3 to 281.4 million). However, during the same period persons older than 55, 65, 75, and 80 more than doubled (from 25.8 to 59.3 million), nearly trebled (from 12.4 to 35 million), more than quadrupled (from 3.9 to 16.6 millions), and more than quintupled (from 1.7 to 9.2 million), respectively (Figure 5-middle frame). Projected aging of the US population through 2100 can be viewed at the US Census Bureau web site [22]. As a result of the aging population, the average life expectancy in the US rose from 62.9 years in 1950 to 76.7 years in 1998. Substantial gains in life expectancy have also occurred in most regions of the world except Sub-Saharan Africa, which accounts for 83% of the world's AIDS deaths, former Soviet Union countries, affected by the collapse of the socio-economic order, and some parts of Central Africa, convulsed by wholesale genocide. Whether such population aging trends are sustainable long term is questionable. While some believe biological limits will cap average life expectancy at approximately 85 years, others view improved nutrition, judicious behavioral and life-style changes, and broad-based access to ever improving medical care as extending average life expectancy well beyond the 100-years mark. The latter scenario is supported by rising rather than plateauing life expectancy in Western Europe and Japan, where it is the highest. In some of these countries life expectancy is rising at a faster rate now than it did in the early 1900s.

Aging increases the risk of developing cancer and approximately 75% of cancers occur in individuals 55 years of age and older [23]. Moreover, the risk rises exponentially with increasing age in both, men and women. For example, the age- and population-adjusted cancer incidence in 2000 was 99 in women ages 30-34 but rose to 270 between ages 40 and 44, 1,080 between 60 and 64, and peaked at 1,926 between 80 and 84 (Figure 5-lower frame). Men's cancer risk increased even more dramatically from 62 between ages 30-34, to 3,160 for men ages 80 to 84 [24]. As a result of the aging US population and other factors, cancer incidence rates rose by an average of 1.2% per year between 1950 and 1997, but by 1.6% for individuals between ages 65 and 74 [25]. Most of the rise can be accounted for by exploding lung cancer incidence rates in American men through 1990 (Figure 2-top), and to a lesser extent in American women (Figure 2-bottom). Likewise, mortality rates rose by 0.2% a year during this 49-year period [26] resulting from rising rates for individuals 65 and older that exceeded more modest declines in mortality rates through age 64. Rising mortality rates paralleled the rise in lung cancer incidence rates, a malignancy associated with a short survival given its tendency to early dissemination and unresponsiveness to present day chemotherapy. Since 1993 mortality rates have decreased modestly, especially for certain cancers. However, these declines have little to do with treatment of cancer per se. More on this later.

In the meantime, baring catastrophic events such as global war or uncontrollable epidemics, the US and world populations will continue to increase and age for the foreseeable future. As a result, increasing numbers of individuals will be at risk of developing cancer and die of their disease unless drastic changes are made in way the *War on Cancer* is conducted.

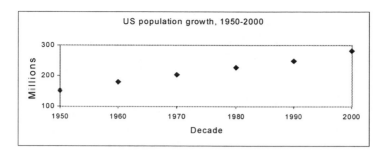

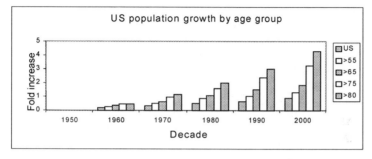

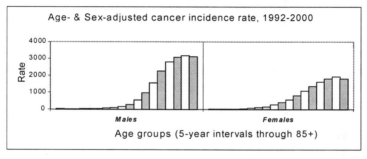

Figure -5. Growth (top) and aging (center) of the US population. Source: National Center for Health Statistics. Health, United States 2004, with chartbook on Trends in the health of Americans. Hyattsville, MD. 2004. Age- and sex-adjusted cancer incidence rates, US 1992-2000 (bottom). Source: Annual Report to the Nation on the Status of Cancer, 1975-2000 (corrections/errata and supplemental information).

PART II

What is cancer?

Chapter 3

CANCER THROUGH THE AGES

Cancer is not a modern-age ailment: it has afflicted humans at all times and in all regions of the world. The first evidence consists of tumor masses found in fossilized human bones from pre-historic times. Cancerous growths have also been found in Egyptian and Peruvian mummies dating back to approximately 1500 BC. The earliest descriptions of what is generally agreed today to have been cancer appeared in ancient Egyptian manuscripts discovered in the 19th century, especially the George Ebers, Edwin Smith, and the Kahun Gynecological papyri, written between 1500 and 1600 BC. The Smith papyrus, in particular, describes solid and ulcerating breast tumors that were treated with a *"fire drill"* [27]. In ancient times, gods were thought to preside over human destiny, including health and disease, medicine and religion were intertwined and practiced by priests and sages, and famous physicians were deified. Following the decline of Egypt, Greek medicine became preeminent, especially with Hippocrates (460-377 BC), whose humor system of health and disease became the foundation of medical care for the ensuing 2000 years.

1.   FROM ANCIENT EGYPT TO GREECE AND ROME

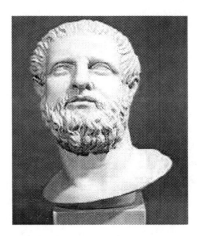

Figure -6. Hippocrates

Hippocrates believed that health resulted from the balance and disease from the imbalance in four body humors: black bile, yellow bile, phlegm, and blood, each originating in a different organ and each matching a physical earthly element and a specific season (Table V). The relative dominance of one of the humors determined personality traits and their imbalance resulted in a propensity to certain diseases. Thus, the aim of treatment was to restore balance through diet, exercise, and the judicious use of herbs, oils, earthly compounds, and occasionally heavy metals or surgery. Hippocrates is known as the *Father of Medicine* more for rejecting the prevailing Aesculapius' view of the supernatural causes of disease, for promoting the rational approach to medicine, and for his famous Oath, rather than for his voluminous 60 books of medical writings. Hippocrates wrote extensively about diseases that produced masses (*onkos*), and coined the word *karkinos* to describe ulcerating and non-healing lumps that in retrospect included lesions ranging from benign processes to malignant tumors. He advocated diet, rest, and exercise for mild illnesses, followed by purgatives, heavy metals and surgery for more serious diseases, especially *karkinomas*. His stepwise treatment approach is summarized in one of his *Aphorisms*. "*What drugs will not cure, the knife will; what the knife will not cure, the cautery will; what the cautery will not cure must be considered incurable*". To his credit, he recognized the relentless progression of deep-seated *karkinomas* and the often-negative effect of treatment when he wrote: "*It is best not to apply any treatment in cases of occult karkinomas for, if treated,the patients die quickly; but if not treated, they hold out for a long time"* (*Aphorism #38 Book 6* [28]). The view that *"the excised karkinomas have returned and caused death"* [29] was also held by Hippocrates' successors including Aulus Cornelius Celsus (30 BC - 50 AD) who wrote, *"Some have applied caustics, cautery, scalpel, or medicines but none have helped"*, and Archigenes (54-117 AD) who advised *"If it has taken anything into its claws it cannot be easily ripped away"* [30].

Table -V. Hippocrates' Humoral system of health and disease.

Humor	Organ	Temperament	Element	Season
Blood	Heart	Sanguine	Air	Spring
Black bile	Spleen	Melancholic	Earth	Summer
Yellow bile	Liver	Choleric	Fire	Fall
Phlegm	Brain	Phlegmatic	Water	Winter

Galen (Clavdii Galeni, 129-210 AD), physician to three Roman emperors, was the second most famous physician of the ancient world and one of the most prolific with his 500 works. He also was a brilliant anatomist and philosopher, and a poet. He bridged the Greek and the Roman medical worlds and enshrined Hippocratic principles as the foundation of all medical knowledge through the Middle Ages. His major contribution to understanding cancer was the classification of tumors into: *tumores secondum naturam* (tumors according to nature) which included physiologic processes such as the growth of breasts during puberty or of the pregnant uterus; *tumores supra naturam* (tumors above nature), such as abscesses or inflammations; and, *tumores praeter naturam* (tumors beyond nature). He subdivided the latter into: *onkoi* (lumps or masses in general), *karkinos* (included malignant ulcers), and *karkinomas* (included non-ulcerating cancers) [31]. Yet, despite his enormous influence on medical practice of the following 1500 years, Galen's original contributions to cancer treatment were minimal.

2. THE MIDDLE AGES: BYZANTIUM, THE MUSLIMS, AND THE PRE-RENAISSANCE

With the collapse of Greco-Roman civilization after the fall of Rome in 476 AD, medical knowledge stagnated and many ancient medical writings were lost. Nevertheless, prominent physicians emerged during the Byzantine Empire at the end of the 4th Century, including Oribasius of Pergamum and Paul of Aegina, both of whom advocated surgery for breast and uterine cancers. At the same time, systematic translations of Greek medical texts into Arabic began by Nestorian monks (a Syrian order affiliated with the

Patriarchy of Constantinople) were continued by Muslim scholars thus ensuring their preservation for posterity. Islamic physician-scholars were the most prominent of this period, including the illustrious and influential Rhazes (864-925), Avicenna (980-1037), and Avenzoar (1091-1161). However, they were not innovators modeling their practice and writings after Hippocratic and Galenic principles. Of interest is Avenzoar (Abu Marwan Abd al-Malik Ibn Zuhr in Arabic, 1091-1161) who first described the symptoms of esophageal cancer, in his book *Kitab al-Taissir*, and proposed feeding enemas to keep alive patients with stomach cancer [32], a treatment approach unsuccessfully attempted by his predecessors. The 9th Century saw the rise of *The Studium* of Salerno, Italy, the first formal associations of scholarly physicians. Fostered by its Greek past, it was sustained by the medical needs of thousands of crusaders en route to Palestine. Although the *Studium* had little direct impact on the progress of medicine it was the precursor to the emergence of the greatly influential pre-Renaissance medical schools at Montpellier (1150), Bologna (1158), and Paris (1208).

3.   FROM THE RENAISSANCE TO WORLD WAR II

The early-Renaissance period witnessed a revival of interest in Greek culture fostered by the arrival in Western Europe of many Greek scholars who fled Constantinople after the Turks conquered Byzantium in 1453, thus enabling western scholars to abandon Arabic translations of the Greek masters. This and other transcendental events of that time, such as the invention of the printing press, the discovery of America, and the Reformation, brought about a change in direction and outlook: a desire to escape the boundaries of the past, and an eagerness to explore new horizons. This inquisitiveness was broad-based, encompassing all areas of human knowledge and endeavor from the study of anatomy to the scrutiny of the skies, and culminated in the publication of two revolutionary and immensely influential treatises of that period: *"De Humani Corporis Fabrica Libri Septum"* (Seven Books on the Fabric of the Human Body) [33] by Andreas Vessalius (1514-1564), and *"De Revolutionibus orbium coelestium* (On the revolutions of the celestial orbs) by Nicolaus Copernicus (1473-1543). Likewise, progress was made in surgical techniques and treatment of wounds, thanks to the Ambroise Paré (1510-1590) [34], the father of modern surgery, whose extensive experience on the battlefields of France's armies and ingenious prostheses reduced surgical mortality and accelerated rehabilitation. However, this burst of Renaissance knowledge did not extend to cancer, leading Paré to call all cancers *Noli me tangere* (do not touch me) and to declare, "*Any kind of cancer is almost incurable and...* (if operated)...*heals with great difficulty*" [35].

Nonetheless, some of the physical attributes of cancer began to emerge. Gabriele Fallopio (1523-1562) is credited to having described the clinical differences between benign and malignant tumors, a distinction largely applicable today. He recognized malignant tumors by their woody firmness, irregular shape, multi-lobulation, adhesion to neighboring tissues (skin, muscles, and bones), and by their surrounding congested blood vessels. In contrast, benign tumors were said to be softer masses of regular shape (often round) that are movable and do not adhere to adjacent structures. He also advocated a cautious approach to cancer treatment, "*Quiescente cancro, medicum quiescentrum*" (If a cancer doesn't bother, leave it alone). More importantly, for the first time in 1500 years the Galen's black bile theory of the origin of cancer was challenged and new hypotheses were formulated. For example, Paracelsus' (Wilhelm Bombast von Hohenheim, 1493-1541) proposed to substitute Galen's black bile by *"ens"* (entities): *ens astrorum* (cosmic entities); *ens veneni* (toxic entities); *ens naturale et spirituale* (physical or mental entities); and *ens deale* (Providential entities). Similarly, Johannes Baptista van Helmont (1577-1644) envisioned a mysterious "*Archeus*" system [36].

While these hypotheses were throwbacks to pre-Hippocratic beliefs in supernatural forces governing human health and disease, it was at this time that René Descartes (1590-1650) published his "*Discours de la méthode pour bien conduire sa raison et chercher la verité dans les sciences*" [36] (Discourse on rightly conducting one's reason for seeking the truth in the sciences). This philosophical treatise on the method of systematic doubt was pivotal in guiding thinkers and researchers in their quest for the truth. Thus, the discovery of chyle (lymph) [38] by Gaspare Aselli (1581-1626) and of its circulation and final drainage into the blood circulation discovered by William Harvey (1578-1657) lead scholars to conclude that Galen's black bile implicated in cancer could be found nowhere, whereas lymph was everywhere and was therefore suspect. Based on this new lead, Henri François Le Dran (1685-1770) hypothesized than cancer began as a local disease best treated with surgery but once spread through lymphatics was inoperable and fatal [39]. His contemporary, Jean-Louis Petit (1674-1750), advocated total mastectomy for breast cancer, including the resection of axillary glands (lymph nodes), which he correctly judged necessary "*to preclude recurrences*" [40,41]. His approach to breast cancer surgery is still current today, albeit with many technical modifications. How lymph might induce cancer was somewhat of a puzzle and several hypotheses were proposed. For example, Bernard Peyrilhe (1735-1804) postulated the presence of an *"Ichorous matter"*, a cancer-promoting factor akin to a virus, emerging from degenerated or putrefied lymph [42]. To test whether the *Ichorous matter* was contagious, he injected cancer fluid from a mammary carcinoma under the skin of a dog, which he kept at home under observation. However, his servants drowned the constantly howling dog thus cutting short the experiment. Peyrilhe was also the first to advance the notion of the local origin of cancer and viewed disease emerging distally as "*consequent cancers*". The term *metastases* to describe these secondary cancers was coined in 1829 by Joseph Recamier, a French gynecologist better known for advocating the use of the vaginal speculum to examine female genitalia. On another front, recognizing that the special needs of cancer patients were not being met, monk Jean Godinot founded the first cancer hospital (*Hopital des cancers*) in 1740, in Reims, France, in the midst of strong protestations by neighborhood inhabitants. It initially welcomed 5 women and 3 men.

In the meantime Bernardino Ramazzini (1633-1714), the father of modern occupational medicine, had produced the first convincing evidence of a link between the environment and human diseases. After years of painstaking observations on the field, he published in 1700 a treatise entitled *De morbis artificum diatriba* (Diseases of workers) listing 52 occupational illnesses [43]. In 1713, he reported a virtual absence of cervical cancer but a high incidence of breast cancer in nuns relative to married women and thought there might be a connection to their celibacy, a notion widely held until challenged in 1991 [44]. Years later (1761), John Hill warned of the dangers of tobacco stating "*No man should venture upon Snuff, who is not sure that he is not so far liable to a cancer: and no man can be sure of that* " [45], and Percivall Pott linked scrotum cancer to chimney sweeping in 1775. Other baffling observations of that time included recurrence at sites distal from the original cancer, multiple cancers in a single individual, and families with a high incidence of cancer. Such occurrences were explained by a certain cancer predisposition or *diathesis* as invoked by Jacques Delpech (1772-1835) and Gaspard Laurent Bayle (1774-1816) [46], and later re-energized throughout Europe by Pierre Paul Broca (1824-1880), Sir James Paget, and Carl von Rokitansky (1804-1878). Followers of the *diathesis* theory viewed cancer as a local manifestation of a constitutional defect. Consequently, they were generally nihilistic regarding therapy as they considered cancer relapses nearly inevitable unless resected very early. However, the observation that at least some cancers were surgically curable, convinced Peyrilhe that cancer is a local disease, and that relapses after surgery are either local re-growth of remnant disease, or unrecognized early dissemination through blood or lymph vessels, as first postulated by Cruveilhier and later amplified by Heinrich von Waldeyer-Hartz (1836-1931), and Franz Konig (1832-1910). The latter proposed a widely embraced pathophysiologic classification of metastases that provided a rational foundation for cancer staging and hence prognosis assessment that endures today. He divided recurrences into three categories: local, regional, and distal, depending on whether the new cancer arose from remnants of the initial cancer incompletely resected, from its spread to lymphatic tissues, or as a result of its distal dissemination through veins, as first observed by Broca [47].

Zaccharias and Hans Jansen had invented a prototype of the microscope, circa 1590. However, many years would pass before powerful and distortion-free (achromatic) instruments, introduced by Vincent Chevalier in the 18th Century, identified cells as the fundamental structural and functional unit of plants and animals, setting the stage for new hypotheses about cancer to emerge. For example, Johannes Muller (1801 - 1858) devoted his efforts to the microscopic study of the disease and in 1839 published "*On the fine structure and forms of morbid tumors*". He postulated than cancer originated, not from normal tissue, but from "*budding elements*" which his 500-fold magnifying microscope failed to identify. Alternatively, Adolf Hannover (1814-1894) fancied that cancer arose from a specific "*cellula cancrosa*" that was different form normal cells in size and appearance. However, Rudolph Virchow (1821-1902) and his followers were unable to confirm the existence of such a cell [48], a view first articulated by Alfred Armand Louis Marie Velpeau (1795-1867). After examining 400 malignant and 100 benign tumors under the microscope Velpeau concluded, as if he had correctly anticipated the genetics bases of cancer, "*The so-called cancer cell is merely a secondary product rather than the essential element in the disease. Beneath it, there must exist some more intimate element which science would need in order to define the nature of cancer*" [49]. Robert Remak (1815-1865) took another step forward by postulating that cancer was not a "*new formation*" but a "*transformation*" of normal tissues, which resembles or, if degeneration ensues, differs from the tissue of origin [50]. This view was expanded by Louis Bard (1829-1894) who proposed, also correctly, that normal cells are capable of developing into a mature, differentiated state, whereas cancer cells suffer from developmental defects that result in tumor formation [51]. Remak's and Bard's notions are significant in that they provide clues on the genetic origin of cancer and served as precursors of today's histologic classification of many cancers into: "*well differentiated*", "*moderately differentiated*", and "*poorly differentiated*" subtypes, a stratification still useful today to plan treatment and to gage prognosis. Another notable scientist, who bridged Velpeau's views on the origin of cancer to our present knowledge, was Theodor Boveri (1862-1915). In an essay entitled "*Zur Frage der Entstehung maligner Tumoren*" [52] (The Origin of malignant tumors), Boveri first proposed a role for somatic mutations in cancer development based on his observation that abnormal fertilization of urchin eggs lead to anomalous cell divisions, chromosomal loss, and the emergence of tissue masses. Thus, it would take 50 years of progress for Boveri to validate Velpeau's intuition, and another half a century for the emergence of molecular biology and molecular genetics to confirm Boveri's initially ignored views on the nature of cancer.

Yet, while small pieces of the cancer puzzle were slowly falling into place, the true nature of cancer and the code governing its development, growth, and dissemination remained a mystery and remedies continued whimsical and inefficacious. Indeed, Oliver Wendell Holmes, addressing the Massachusetts Medical Society in 1860, summed up the status of drugs at the time: *"If the whole materia medica, as now used, could be sunk to the bottom of the sea, it would be all the better for mankind – and all the worse for the fishes"* [53]. As this statement resonated in America, progress in bacteriology and parasitology was having a profound impact on cancer theory and cancer therapeutics of the 19th century. Interest in a possible bacterial or parasitic link to cancer, first raised in the 17th and 18th century, lead to equating cancer invasion to bacterial infections and adopting the bacteria-eradication concept as a goal for treating cancer, a notion that still prevails today. Between the 1880's and the 1920's, the hunt for cancer-causing microorganisms was obstinate and relentless as summed up by S.Peller [54], *"every conceivable group of microorganisms was the search target: worms, bacilli, cocci, spirochetes; molds, fungi, coccidiae; sporozoa, ameba, trypanosomas; polimorphous microorganisms, and filtrable viruses. It was like fishing in a well-stocked pond. Most fishermen became victims of self-deception..."*.

The zenith of this particular saga was reached when Johannes Andreas Grib Fibiger was awarded the 1926 Nobel Prize in Physiology or Medicine, *"for his discovery of the Spiroptera carcinoma"*. In the presentation speech [55], the Dean of the Royal Caroline Institute stated *"By feeding healthy mice with cockroaches containing the larvae of the spiroptera, Fibiger succeeded in producing cancerous growths in the stomachs of a large number of animals. It was therefore possible, for the first time, to change by experiment normal cells into cells having all the terrible properties of cancer"*. The hypothesis of the transmissibility of cancer that endured several decades is of historical interest as it exemplifies how an entire generation of scientists and scholars, misguided by flawed hypotheses, often commit their talents and energy, as well as human and financial resources in the unproductive pursuit of a false lead. While the determined pursuit of a worthy goal by many is often necessary, overly enthusiastic adherence to a single hypothesis by many is self-reinforcing and can obfuscate good judgment while rejecting the unwelcome views of isolated dissenters. The hypothesis of the bacteriological basis of cancer eventually lost its luster, but not before it had established another, more pervasive and counterproductive, parallel with infectious diseases: that cancer cells, like bacteria, are foreign invaders that must be eradicated at any cost. In turn, this has lead to the development of ever more powerful cytotoxic drugs and increasingly aggressive treatment regimens but few cures. Another legacy of this period is a drug development strategy by trial and error, pioneered by Ehrlich in his 7-year quest for anti-microbials, a simplistic approach not suited for cancer drug development that unjustifiably persists today, as discussed in Chapter 6. Finally, 150 years later and based of inconclusive evidence, the cancer-bacteria link is being revived by implicating the bacterium *"Helicobacter pylori"*, in the genesis of gastric carcinoma [56] and MALT, a low-grade non-Hodgkin's Lymphoma, leading the International Agency for Research on Cancer to classify *H. pylori* as a Group 1 human carcinogen, in 1994. However, recent data suggest that MALT might straddle between malignancy and inflammation [57]

The discovery of anesthesia in 1842 by Crawford W Long [58] and of asepsis in 1867 by Joseph Lister [59] propelled surgery to the forefront of early-stage cancer management. Likewise, the discovery of X-rays by Wilhelm Conrad Roentgen in 1895 [60] and of radium by Marie and Pierre Curie in 1896 [60] marked the dawn of modern diagnostic and therapeutic radiology and of nuclear medicine. In contrast, treatment of advanced-stage cancer was inefficacious at best and harmful at worst, and the lives of patients with disseminated cancer continued to be wretched and short. Indeed, centuries-old cancer remedies were used through the middle of the 20th Century, including herbs, plants, and salts of heavy metals, such as mercury, lead, iron, copper, gold, and mostly arsenic in powder or paste form. The inefficacy of these mainstream agents set the stage for the proliferation of alternate treatment approaches often promoted by charlatans making farfetched claims, as is usually the case.

Some of the most outlandish treatments of the 18th Century include the *"Storck"* and the *"lagartija"* cures. Anton Storck, a Viennese physician, claimed that a hemlock concoction of his own making was highly effective against breast and uterine cancers when administered in sufficiently high doses to cause faintness (his version of today's *"toxicity-limiting"* dosing approach). A colorful example of the extraordinary gullibility of physicians and the public alike followed a publication, in 1783, by a Guatemalan university professor praising the curative properties of a Central American *lagartija* (lizard) [61]. This particular lizard could cure venereal diseases, leprosy, and cancer. The lizards had to be beheaded, skinned, disemboweled, and swallowed whole. The prescribed dose was one lizard the first day, two the next, and so on until nausea became intolerable (his version of today's *"maximum tolerated dose"* chemotherapy). In such cases, animals could be sliced into small pieces to make the remedy more palatable and patients more compliant. The exotic nature and origin of this treatment, its peculiar formulation and dosing schedule, and the fact that it was shrouded in the mystique of an old American Indian remedy contributed to its immediate success and enthusiastic acceptance throughout Europe. It was the subject of innumerable medical testimonials, several books and reports in French, Italian, and German, and of at least one doctoral thesis before it finally vanished into oblivion half a century later.

In the absence of cancer treatment breakthroughs, alternate approaches continued through the 19th Century. Two of the most popular were the *"cura famis"* and *"treatment by cold"*. These are of interest to us because, although they rallied few patrons at the time, they resurfaced in the late twentieth century justified by advances in molecular biology and biotechnology of our time. The *cura famis,* or cure by hunger, consisted of starving the cancer through a water diet that could last up to 40 or 50 days. However, patient non-compliance and its ineffectiveness lead to a more radical variant: the severing of the cancer's blood supply. The idea is attributed to William Harvey who observed that ligation of afferent testicular arteries, to deprive the testis of nutrients, resulted in testicular atrophy and necrosis [62]. However, testicular cancer was the only natural target for such an approach given its anatomy that facilitated access to feeding vessels, and the procedure never caught on, despite its well-founded if simplistic rationale. One and a half centuries later, *cura famis* and its variant reappeared under the new name of *"angiogenesis inhibition"*, or the starving of tumors using biological agents that inhibit new vessel formation necessary for cancer growth [63]. The *treatment by cold,* proposed by Scottish surgeon John Hughes Bennett (1821-1875), was the application of cold which he described as *"one of the most powerful means we have to slow the progress of cancer"* [64]. Ironically, that same year he questioned the validity of Pasteur's pivotal experiments refuting spontaneous generation. Bennett's method consisted of applying a mixture of two parts of chopped ice and one part of sea salt to the tumor for 15 to 20 minutes, each week [65]. Although this treatment had no effect on cancer progression, it seemed to alleviate pain. It is worth mentioning that although this method never achieved any degree of success, the concept resurfaced at the end of the twentieth century in the form of heat and hypoxia used as an adjunct to chemotherapy in futile attempts to enhance the susceptibility of cancer cells to the cytotoxicity of cancer drugs [66]. Heat or cold were delivered during surgery (*"thermo-* or *cryo-surgery"*), under magnetic resonance imaging guidance, to treat drug-resistant cancers especially in anatomically-inaccessible sites such as liver metastases [67,68].

During the early part of the 20th century, medical researchers systematically explored different theories of the nature and origin of cancer, leading to incremental progress on many fronts. For example, John Hill's suspicion in 1761 that tobacco had induced nose cancers in heavy snuffers and Percivall Pot's 1775 suggestion of a tar-cancer link in chimney sweepers, were confirmed in 1915 when Katsusaburo Yamagiwa demonstrated that painting rabbits' skin with tar, repeatedly and over long periods, induced cancer. Likewise, the virus-cancer link was confirmed in 1911 when Peyton Rous was able to induce cancer in healthy chickens by injecting them with a cell-free extract of the tumor of a sick chicken. Rous' findings were rejected by much of the medical establishment for they challenged the prevailing view of the genetic heredity of cancer, and he was ostracized for many years. Fifty years later he was awarded the Nobel Prize for Physiology or Medicine for his momentous discovery. Aided by new experimental techniques, more powerful research instruments, and by the compilation of cancer incidence and mortality data, the carcinogenicity of radiation, tobacco, sunlight, and of certain chemical agents was established. As these risks and other aspects of cancer became known, growing public awareness and interest triggered a response by policy makers which eventually prompted the US Congress to enact the National Cancer Act of 1937, the first major attempt to address cancer at the national level.

However, the first human study objectively demonstrating the anti-cancer effect of a drug, albeit very modest, took place during World War II while the origin and nature of cancer remained shrouded in mystery through the middle of the twentieth century when critical advances in biological sciences and in biotechnology began to uncover its genetic basis, discussed in the next Chapter.

Chapter 4

OUR CURRENT UNDERSTANDING

1.   THE GENETIC BASIS OF CANCER

1.1   First the basics

Cancer is not one disease but an assortment of over 200 diverse diseases that can arise from all tissues and organs. For example, cancers arising from blood cells are called *leukemias*; those arising from organ tissues such as the liver or the lungs are called *solid* tumors. More than one type of cancer can originate from an organ or tissue, as is the case of *Lymphomas*, a group of malignancies of the lymphatic system, encompassing more than 20 related cancers, depending on the classification used [69,70]. Cancers can exhibit slow growth patterns compatible with long and symptom-free survival, such as indolent lymphomas or chronic lymphocytic leukemia [71,72], or can quickly progress causing symptoms and death in only a few months, as is the case of acute myelocytic leukemia and pancreatic cancer [73]. Likewise, some cancers quickly spread distally from the site of origin, such as colon, prostate, and lung cancer that often reach liver, bone, and brain, respectively. Others tend to invade locally as is the case of head and neck cancers. Yet, despite their heterogeneous origin, distinct clinical features, and vastly different course and outcome, the underlying genetic processes leading to their development, growth, and dissemination are similar.

The master blueprint that determines the structure and function of all organisms, including man, is called the *"genome"*. Each of the approximately 30 trillion cells that make a human being contains a copy of the entire genome and its approximately 30,000 *"genes"*, neatly packaged in 46 microscopic units called *"chromosomes"* found bundled in the cell *"nucleus"*. Genes are deoxyribonucleic acid (DNA) sequences that contain the code for cells to produce proteins, which are the signals that control the structure and function of each cell, of each organ, and ultimately of the entire organism. These cell-produced, cell-targeted protein signals are at the center of the interdependent relationship that characterizes both the harmonious function of normal cells, and the aberrant behavior of cancer cells. Thus, the genome can be thought of as the book of life where chromosomes are chapters and genes are the carefully crafted sentences made of precise words spelled with "*nucleotide bases*", all sequentially arranged on the DNA molecule. During the process of cell division and of human reproduction the entire genome must be duplicated and passed from cell to cell and from parent to offspring. While this process is prodigiously accurate, *"spelling"* errors do occur. Minor alterations are corrected by *"DNA repair"* genes. Major errors activate "*gate-keeper*" genes that block cell replication and force the cell to commit suicide (*"apoptosis"*). The role of DNA repair and gate-keeper genes is to ensure genomic integrity as cells advance through their replication cycle (*"cell cycle"*). However, occasional non-lethal alterations escape detection, repair, or blockade and are transmitted from a replicating cell to its daughter cells. Transmitted alterations of DNA sequences outside of genes, called *"polymorphism"*, are neither beneficial nor harmful to the cell or the host. Conversely, transmitted alterations within gene sequences, called *"mutations"*, are responsible for approximately 4,000 human diseases, including cancer. When mutations affect an egg or a sperm, they can be transmitted to future generations, resulting in familial predisposition to diseases such as hemophilia, and to some cancers such as retinoblastoma. At present, the genetic fingerprints of most cancers are not known mainly because insensitive detection techniques of the pre-genomic era uncovered mostly structural chromosomal abnormalities visible by light microscopy that are seldom disease-specific. While diagnostically and prognostically valuable in the clinical setting, such gross abnormalities seldom provide insight into the genetic defects responsible for the development, growth, and dissemination of cancer.

Recognizing that the genome occupied a central role in health and disease, the US Department of Energy's Health and Environmental Research Advisory Group recommended, in 1987, launching a "*15-year, multidisciplinary, scientific, and technological undertaking to map and sequence the human genome*". A year later the National Institutes of Health received congressional authority and funding to coordinate and support genomics activities in cooperation with other federal agencies, academia, and international groups. An independent NIH institute, named The National

Human Genome Research Institute, was created to that effect. The overall goal was to identify the position and sequence of the 3-billion nucleotide bases (*letters*) that make up the human genome. However, because the book of life is written as a continuous string of sequential letters without separation or punctuation between words, sentences or paragraphs, deciphering the position and sequence of the nucleotide bases would still be unreadable and uninterpretable. Thus, another major goal was to identify all human genes (the *"words"* and *"sentences"* made up of strings of *"letters"*) and determine their location. The project formally began in 1990, cosponsored by the U.S. Department of Energy and the National Institutes of Health, as a $3 billion, 15-year effort. The first 5-year plan, intended to guide research between 1990 and 1995, was revised in 1993 due to unexpected progress. The second and the third and final 5-year plans outlined goals through 1998 and 2003, respectively.

At present 18 countries participate in the worldwide effort, with significant contributions from research centers in the United Kingdom, Germany, France, and Japan. In direct competition with this multinational group of government and academic research centers arose Celera Genomics. This was a publicly owned biotechnology company established in May 1998 by the PE Corporation and J. Craig Venter, Ph.D., founder of The Institute for Genomic Research at the NIH. Using a faster DNA sequencing strategy, known as the *"whole-genome shotgun"* method, and highly automated sequencing machines that require human attention only 15 minutes per day despite running continuously, Celera (*"swift"* in Latin) was able to publish, in February 2001, a working draft of the human genome sequence [74]. The same month, the Human Genome Project published its own draft, ten years in the making [75]. The human genome sequence was completed in April 2003. However, years will pass before this information is translated into tangible medical benefits for they will require uncovering the genetic bases of disease and designing targeted drugs to prevent, reverse, or control the defective genes or modulate their encoded protein products. In the meantime, government- and industry-sponsored initiatives have made substantial progress, particularly accelerated DNA sequencing, and gene identification and mapping. For example, while it took 9 years for Dr. Lap-Chee Tsui's team to discover the cystic fibrosis gene in 1989 [76], the Parkinson's disease gene was mapped in only 9 days by Dr. Robert Nussbaum's team 9 years later [77].

Thus, the post-genomic era is poised to uncover the genetic defects that render normal cells malignant, and exploit that knowledge for designing agents suitable to reverse or control the genetic defects responsible for the development, growth, and dissemination of cancer. Details of our current knowledge underlying cancer are described next. Readers not especially interested in the details of cancer genetics can omit that section and advance to section *How does cancer arise?* starting on page 53.

1.2   More details

1.2.1   DNA

On March 7th, 1953, Francis Crick, a 35-year old graduate student at the Cavendish laboratory of the University of Cambridge, England, walked into the Eagle pub and declared, "*we* (along with James Watson) *have found the secret of life*". He was referring to their discovering the structure of DNA that explained transmission of genetic information from cell to cell and from parent to offspring, and helped understand how genetic mutations are produced. Theirs was a brilliant interpretation of other investigators' published and, reportedly, unpublished research data. Crick's career had evolved from physics to chemistry and biology. The 23-year old Watson had received a B.S degree from the University of Chicago and a Ph.D. degree in zoology from Indiana University. However, as a research fellow at the Cavendish laboratory, he abandoned his chosen field for "*the pursuit of glory*", as he recounts in his memoirs entitled "*The double Helix: A personal account of the discovery of the structure of DNA*" [78]. In that book, he described his obsession with the DNA molecule and his anticipation that unraveling its structure would bring the Nobel Prize. After attending a 1951 lecture where the gifted Rosalind Franklin presented X-ray crystallography data and her helical concept of the DNA molecule, Watson and Crick built a three-chain DNA molecule model with the backbone on the inside that drew sharp criticism. The head of the Cavendish laboratory, Sir Lawrence Bragg, ordered the pair to leave DNA to King's College where Franklin and her rival Maurice Wilkins were assigned the task. However, when Linus Pauling, a brilliant American chemist, published a wrong structure for DNA, it became evident to them someone else might succeed in winning "*the most important of all scientific prizes*" [78]. According to a special report published on August 17, 1998 in U.S. News [79] "*When Watson came calling in January 1953, Wilkins* (described in Watson's book [78] as '*a beginner in X-ray diffraction work, wanted some professional help and hoped that 'Rosy', a trained crystallographer, could speed up his research'), revealed he had been quietly copying Franklin's data. He showed one of her x-ray photos*". Watson was so impressed that he later wrote "*The instant I saw the picture my mouth fell open and my pulse began to race.... the black cross of reflections which dominated the picture could arise only from a helical structure... mere inspection of the X-ray picture gave several of the vital helical parameters"* [78]. Watson's own admission, the fact that neither he nor Crick conducted research on DNA, relying instead on other investigators' data to draw diagrams and construct tri-dimensional models, and the short time between this episode and the publication of their report leads to the inescapable conclusion: Franklin's photo was pivotal in their inferring the correct molecular structure of DNA. Their highly acclaimed and universally accepted model included two helical chains made of sugar-phosphate backbones, as Franklin's work revealed, held together by complementary pairs of four nitrogen bases interlocked between them. Thus, Watson's and Crick's failure to acknowledge Franklin's crucial role in their formulation of the structure of DNA in the April 2, 1953 *Nature* article [80] where he and Crick disclosed their model is a regrettable episode in the annals of great discoveries. To add insult to injury, Watson ridiculed Franklin in his book [78]: *"So it was quite easy to imagine her the product of an unsatisfied mother who unduly stressed the desirability of professional careers that could save bright girls from marriages to dull men"*. Franklin's biographer [81] adds *"'Rosy' was depicted as an aggressive, perhaps belligerent, female subordinate with no respect for her superiors"* who *"refused to think of herself as an assistant to Wilkins"*. Crick, Watson and Wilkins received the 1962 Nobel Prize for Physiology or Medicine. Watson went on to receive the most honors and recognition, including honorary degrees from 22 universities. Franklin died of ovarian cancer in 1958, age 37.

From an anatomical standpoint, the genome is contained in tightly coiled strands of DNA organized in chromosomes, which are housed in the cell nucleus. To illustrate the minuscule size of the DNA, suffice it to say that if unwound the DNA of a single cell (1 million cells fit on the head of a pin) would stretch 5 feet but would be only 50 trillionth of an inch wide. Stretching all the DNA of a human being would reach the sun and back. A human DNA molecule (Figure 7) consists of two strands that wrap around each other like a twisted ladder or a spiral staircase, the so called *"double helix"*, whose sugar and phosphate sides connect to each other by rungs of nitrogen-containing chemicals called *"bases"*. Each strand is a linearly repeated sequence called *"nucleotides"*, made of one sugar, one phosphate, and one nitrogenous base. There are four different bases: adenine (A), thymine (T), cytosine (C), and guanine (G). The order of the bases along the sugar-phosphate backbone, called the DNA sequence, is like a barcode that encrypts the genetic instructions necessary for the structural and functional integrity of an organism with its unique traits. Weak bonds between bases forming base pairs, of which there are approximately 3 billion in the human genome, hold the two DNA strands together. Each time a cell divides its genome is duplicated by DNA replication, a complex process initiated by

DNA polymerase, an enzyme that breaks the weak bonds between base pairs unwinding the *helix* to allow separation of the two DNA strands. Once separated, each strand directs the synthesis of a complementary DNA strand, including matching bases following strict base pairing: adenine with thymine (A-T pair) and cytosine with guanine (C-G pair). Each daughter cell receives one parental and one new DNA strand, thus minimizing chances of errors (mutations) in gene transfer. At the functional cell level, genetic information encoded in nuclear DNA ultimately leads to production of regulatory proteins in the cell cytoplasm. This process requires an intermediary molecule, called ribonucleic acid (RNA). RNA polymerase first "*unzips*" a section of nuclear DNA and copies (transcribes), base-by-base, a given sequence of exposed bases, and moves into the cell cytoplasm as messenger RNA (mRNA) where it translates the genetic code (or message) into synthesis of the particular protein encoded in the exposed DNA.

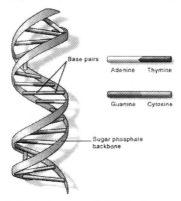

Figure -7. Proposed double-helix structure of DNA. Source: US National Library of Medicine, http://ghr.nlm.nih.gov/dynamicImages/understandGenetics/basics? *DNA.jpg.*

1.2.2   Genes

Johann Mendel entered the Augustinian monastery at Brünn, Moravia (Brno in today's Czech Republic) in 1843, taking the name Gregor. He worked on the side as a substitute teacher in a secondary school in Znaim, near Brünn, and tried to upgrade to regular teacher but failed the certification examination. Ironically, his lowest mark was in biology. His bishop sent him to the University of Vienna for two years to study physics, chemistry mathematics, zoology and botany. However, he never succeeded in passing the examination for a teacher's license. Yet, from his modest monastery garden Mendel unraveled the secrets of heredity. Although he worked alone, Mendel did not operate in a vacuum, for his scientific interests and pursuits were supported by good libraries at the monastery and the school, and by colleagues at the Brünn's Natural Science Society. His now famous description of the experiments that lead to his enlightened conclusions on heredity were presented orally before the Society in 1865, and published in the Society's transactions in 1866 as an article entitled "*Versuche über pflanzenhybriden*" (Experiments with plant hybrids).

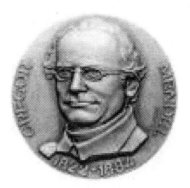

Figure - 8. Gregor Mendel

Mendel crossed several varieties of garden peas by placing pollen from one plant on the female flowers of another, and painstakingly recorded the results. His first major observation contradicted the then popular notion known as "*blending inheritance*" that assumed that all traits were inherited by the offspring as a blend or average of the parents'. Thus, crossing a tall plant with a short one, for example, was expected to produce a medium-sized offspring plant. When Mendel pollinated tall or short plants within themselves, offspring plants remained tall or short, as expected. Curiously, when he cross-pollinated plants with green pea pods with plants that had yellow pods, he noticed that all offspring hybrid plants exhibited green pea pods, as if the yellow pea pod trait had vanished. Yet, when he pollinated two hybrid plants between themselves some of their offspring exhibited yellow pods and others had green pods. Mendel correctly concluded that hereditary traits are discrete packets or particles that pass unchanged from one generation to the next, although each trait might not be expressed in each generation. He called these packets "*elemente*" (elements), and called "*dominant*" those elements that appeared in the offspring and "*recessive*" those that were hidden in the first generation but re-surfaced in the second. He further concluded, also correctly, that paired traits pass from one generation to the next as separate and independent elements. While genetics, particularly human genetics, is more complex with one trait generally being influenced by several genes, and by environmental factors, Mendel's concept of elements, that we call today "*alleles*", and his notion that elements are "*paired*" and inherited as "*separate*" and "*independent*" entities from one another in a "*dominant*" or "*recessive*" fashion, remain largely accurate. Mendel's work fell into oblivion until 1900 when it was re-discovered by botanist William Bateson who became a fervent advocate of Mendel's ideas.

Genes are the fundamental physical and functional units of heredity that are passed from parent to offspring. They are made of specific sequences of DNA bases located on a particular chromosome that encode (contain information for) the production of specific proteins that serve as cellular signals. The size of genes varies widely, from approximately 10,000 to 150,000 base-pairs. However, only a fraction (10%) of the 3 billion base-pairs that constitute the genome represents protein-encoding sequences (*exons*) of genes, the rest being intercalated sequences (*introns*) with no known coding function. Additionally, only a small fraction of the approximately 30,000 human genes are "*expressed*" in any particular cell. For example, hemoglobin genes are expressed in red blood cell precursors, not in muscle or brain cells. Yet, the very presence of all genes in every cell makes each of them a potential source for cloning under the right conditions.

Gene expression begins with the synthesis of an RNA copy *("transcription")* of the DNA gene sequence, in the nucleus, followed by its transport (the RNA becoming messenger RNA or mRNA) to ribosomes, in the cytoplasm, where the encoded genetic information is "*translated*" to protein synthesis. However, before moving to the cytoplasm, non-functional *introns* are snipped out and *exons* are spliced (linked) together, thus giving rise to the proper protein-encoding sequences. Once in the cell cytoplasm, the mRNA serves as a template to translate the encoded information (*codons*) into a string of individual amino acids that constitute the building blocks of protein synthesis. Codons are sequences of three DNA bases within exons that direct cells to produce a specific amino acid. For example, the sequence *ATG* codes for the amino acid methionine. There are 64 possible codons encoding 20 amino acids, thus allowing for code redundancy for all but 2 amino acids: methionine (*AUG*) and tryptophan (*UGG*). The other 18 amino acids are encoded by 2 to 6 codons. For example, *AAA* and *AAG* translate into lysine and *UCU, UCC, UCA, UCG, AGU,* and *AGC* translate into serine. In addition, there is an "*initiation codon*", usually *AUG,* that initiates translation of mRNA, and a "*termination codon*", usually *UAA, UGA* or *UAG*, that ends it. Thus, when the RNA "*reads*" a gene sequence it is prompted where to start and where to end the transcription process. Hence, from a logistic point of view the genetic code is a series of codons, contained in genes in turn housed in chromosomes located in the cell nucleus, that specify which amino acids will be synthesized and in what order. The 20 amino acids, assembled in a variety of different combinations and lengths, give rise to approximately 100,000 proteins encoded in the human genome that are necessary to maintain the structural and functional integrity of human beings. Errors in DNA or RNA transcription, and exon splicing can result in mutations, which in turn can lead to a faulty "*translation*" of the gene code, including failure to synthesize the gene-encoded protein or production of an aberrant protein. The outcome of either will be a functional disruption of the protein-targeted cell.

1.2.3   Chromosomes

Chromosomes house all genes. Thus, it might be expected that the number of chromosomes would increase with increasing complexity of the organism according to an evolutionary scheme. However, this is not the case. While a humble bacterium might function with a single chromosome and mosquitoes need 6, humans have 46, dogs have 78, and goldfish have an unexpected 94. The 46 human chromosomes are organized in two sets of 23 pairs (Figure 9): 22 "*autosomal*" (numbered 1 through 22) and 1 "*sex*" chromosome (X for female and Y for male). Except for the sex chromosomes that determine gender and are thus distinct and different, each set bears identical copies of the entire human genome, and is inherited: one copy from the father and the other from the mother as a result of sexual reproduction. Indeed, germ cells or gonads (spermatozoid or sperm for short in males, ovum or egg in females) contain only one set of 23 chromosomes: 22X in a female ovum, and 22Y or 22X in a male sperm. During reproduction the male sperm delivers its entire genetic load, either 22X or 22Y, into the female egg so that the fertilized egg. Thus, the offspring will contain two identical and complementary sets of 22 chromosomes plus the sex chromosome pair that determines gender: 44XX for female and 44XY for male. In women, one X chromosome is inherited from each parent, whereas in men the X-chromosome derives from the mother and the Y chromosome from the father, who therefore is the parent that determines the gender of the offspring whether male or female.

Genetic alterations or mutations are associated with over 4,000 human diseases including cancer and have been mapped to specific chromosomes [82]. Alterations of any of the 22 *autosomal* chromosomes are associated with *autosomal* diseases, such as sickle cell anemia. Aberrations in *sex* chromosomes (X or Y) lead to sex-linked diseases such as hemophilia A. Genetic alterations involving major structural chromosomal abnormalities, such as multiple copies of a chromosome (as seen in Down syndrome), translocation of part of a chromosome to another (as occurs in Burkitt's lymphoma), or deletions of chromosome or parts thereof (exemplified by the DiGeorge syndrome), are visually detectable under the microscope. This is because appropriately stained chromosomes acquire light and dark transverse bands (reflecting variations in amounts of A-T or G-C base pairs) that enable cytogeneticists to identify each individual chromosome (Figure 9), and recognize structural abnormalities [83]. This test, called chromosome banding, is used routinely in the clinical setting. More subtle defects can now be detected via more sophisticated approaches, including molecular techniques.

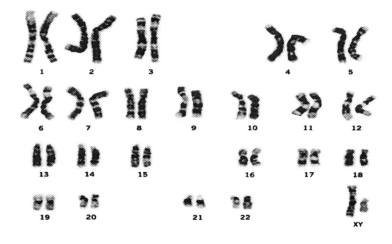

Figure -9. G-banded human male chromosome grouped and numbered according to standard karyotyping practice. Courtesy of Dr. K. Satya-Prakash.

Chromosomal analysis is valuable in cancer management because some cancers, especially hematologic malignancies, harbor structural chromosomal abnormalities that have diagnostic or prognostic significance. A small number of chromosomal abnormalities are virtually diagnostic by themselves. They include, t(9;22), the hallmark of chronic myelocytic leukemia (CML) (Figure 10), shared by a small subset of acute lymphocytic leukemia (ALL), and t(15;17), an abnormality that is specific for acute promyelocytic leukemia. More importantly, the recognition that the t(9;22) translocation confers a growth advantage to CML cells lead to the development of Imatinib mesylate (Gleevec ®), the first successful post-genomic molecularly targeted agent to control rather kill the malignant cells. However, most cancers exhibit either no chromosomal abnormalities detectable by current methodology, as is the case of most solid tumors, or exhibit non-specific but diagnostically and prognostically helpful abnormalities, as is the case of most hematologic malignancies. Examples of these include gene translocations such as t(14;18) in follicular-type non-Hodgkin's lymphoma, t(8;14) in Burkitt's lymphoma, trisomy 12 (three copies of chromosome 12) in chronic lymphocytic leukemia, and del(16)(q22) in a subset of acute myelocytic leukemia.

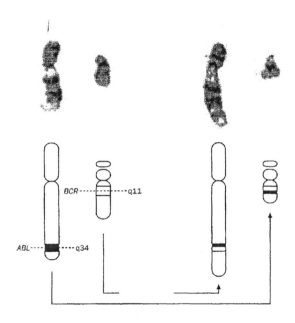

Figure -10. Chromosomal translocation in chronic myelogenous leukemia. The reciprocal translocation between the long arms of chromosomes 9 & 22, which occurs below break points q34 and q11, respectively, are shown on the ideograms (lower panel). Actual chromosomes 9 & 22 from a normal individual (left) and from a patient with chronic myelogenous leukemia (right) are shown in the upper panel. Courtesy of Dr. Avery A. Sandberg.

Additionally, many genetic aberrations are sub-microscopic, precluding their visual detection by chromosomal banding. Such cases can be unmasked by more powerful techniques that use DNA probes such as FISH analyses [84], comparative genomic hybridization [85], spectral karyotyping [86], or recombinant DNA techniques [87]. One example is point mutations that characterize certain hemoglobinopathies (abnormal hemoglobins), where single amino acid substitutions occur on one of the four hemoglobin chains. To illustrate, sickle cell disease and hemoglobin C, two hemoglobinopathies with different symptoms, clinical profiles, and prognoses, result when glutamic acid on position 6 of the β chain is replaced by valine or lysine, respectively.

1.2.4   The cell cycle

Cells undergo two fundamentally different but complementary processes: cell division and cell differentiation. Cell division, which occurs via the cell cycle, ensures self-renewal of undifferentiated precursor cells. In contrast, cell differentiation is designed to generate highly specialized non-dividing cells with distinct and varied functions. Together, these genetically controlled cell processes sustain the structural and functional integrity of the entire organism and ensure genetic transfer to the next generation. For example, bone marrow stem cells possess the ability to divide thus ensuring a constant pool of self-renewing precursor cells. However, they also give rise to a diversity of progenitor cells that, while loosing self-renewing potential, undergo differentiation into the various types of highly specialized blood cells. These include red cells to ensure oxygen delivery to all tissues, white cells to seek, engulf and kill invading microorganisms, and platelets to instantly plug any vascular leak as our first line of defense against accidental blood loss. The cell cycle is divided into several phases (Figure 11): M-phase ("*mitosis*" or cell division), S-phase (DNA synthesis), and G_1 and G_2, the gaps between M and S, and between S and M, respectively. Additionally, cells out of cycle are said to be quiescent or in G_0 and require external stimuli to move them out of G_0 and into G_1. As a cell is triggered by extra-cellular stimuli to go through the cell cycle, it is subjected to a series of checkpoints that ensure the integrity of the DNA and prevents damaged DNA from being passed to daughter cells.

These steps are under the control of numerous genes that promote or inhibit the cell cycle depending on whether or not defective DNA-carrying cells must be repaired or eliminated. Of these, *RB1* and *TP53* are considered the main cell-cycle "*gate-keepers*" through the activity of their encoded proteins, *pRB* and *p53*. Their role is exerted through the *E2F*, a protein that acts as a transcription factor that promotes cell-cycle progression from G1 to S. In normal cells, *E2F* is inhibited by *pRB,* which in turn can be temporarily inactivated by cyclin-dependent kinases of the *m2m* gene product. In cancer cells, *pRB* is inactivated by several mechanisms including loss of function, mutations, and by viral oncogenes, enabling *E2F*-driven excessive cancer cell proliferation. *p53, a* protein encoded by tumor suppressor gene *TP53* (located at 17p13.1), is believed to have a far-reaching role and is sometimes called the *"guardian of the genome"*. It includes activation of genes that control the cell cycle (*WAF1* and *CIP1/p21*), DNA damage repair (*GADD45*), G1 to S and G2 to M progression (*14-3-σ*), and *"apoptosis"* or "*programmed cell death*" (*BAX*). Loss of the latter function is generally viewed as a common pathway in carcinogenesis. *TP53* is the most frequently mutated gene in human somatic cancers, and is responsible for the Li-

Fraumeni syndrome, a rare inherited condition associated with a high risk for developing sarcomas, brain tumors, breast cancer, and leukemias.

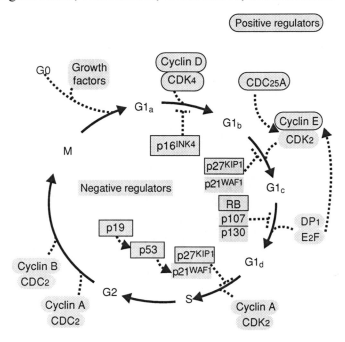

Figure -11. Cell cycle regulation. Positive and negative regulator proteins are identified within oblong and rectangular boxes, respectively. Their points of action at various phases of the cell cycle and their interactions are identified by dotted lines. Reproduced with permission, courtesy of Dr. S. Collins.

1.2.5 Programmed cell death

Like organisms, cells are born, live and die. Also like organisms, cells can die of "*natural*" or "*accidental*" causes. Accidental cell death is caused by a sudden external attack by noxious agents, such as exposure to heat or acid, against which cells play an entirely passive role. In contrast, natural cell death results from a highly complex and genetically controlled process called *programmed cell death* or *apoptosis*. Cell survival is also controlled by a stretch of DNA located at the end of each chromosome, called *"telomeres"*. These two pathways to cell death control cells' life span through distinct though complementary mechanisms. Apoptosis occurs when a cell commits "*suicide*" in response to external signals that challenge and ultimately defeat their self-preservation mechanisms. In contrast, telomere-triggered cell death originates from within the cell as a mechanism that inherently limits its life span and by extension controls aging of the entire organism.

Apoptosis

Unless counterbalanced, cell division would result in the accumulation of so many cells that our body weight and size would nearly double each year. The necessary counterbalance is achieved by desquamation or sloughing off of superficial layers of skin cells and of cells lining hollow organs such as the gastrointestinal, respiratory, and genitourinary tracts, and via apoptosis. Unlike "*accidental*" cell death, a process caused by an acute injury that destroys the cell, spills its content, and triggers an inflammatory response, apoptosis can be viewed as a cell implosion from within, with rapid clearing of cell debris by specialized cells called *"macrophages"*, without causing inflammation. This implosion results from the prevailing effect of genes that promote cell death over the counteracting effects of genes that block it. Apoptotic genes belong to the *BCL-2* gene family encoding at least 14 proteins that promote apoptosis, such as Bax, Bcl-Xs, Bad, Hrk, Bim, Bik, Blk, APR/Noxa, and Bcl-Gs, or block it including BCL-2, Bcl-XL, Bcl-W, Mcl-1, Boo/Diva, and Al/Bff-1. The interaction of these proteins bound to each other determines whether the resulting pair (dimer) promotes or blocks apoptosis. For example, the Bax/Bax and Bcl-2/Bad dimers promote cell death whereas Bax/Bcl-2 and Bcl-2/Bcl-2 dimers protect against it. A myriad of triggers can initiate the apoptotic pathway including chemotherapy drugs, ultraviolet and gamma irradiation, oxidative agents, certain viruses, and cytokines (cell-secreted intercellular mediator proteins). Once initiated the apoptotic mechanism culminates in the activation of a family of cysteine proteases (enzymes that break up proteins) called caspases that by cleaving a variety of cytoplasmic, nuclear, and membrane proteins execute the final steps of the cell death pathway (Figure 12).

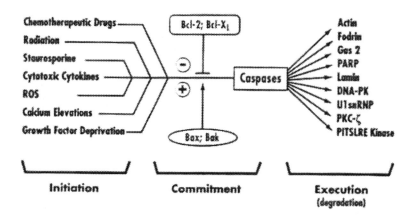

Figure -12. The apoptosis pathway: Reproduced with permission from Dr. JC Reed, Adv Leuk & Lymphoma 7:1997/1998.

The *BCL-2* was discovered in 1985 because of its involvement in chromosome translocation t(14;18) that was found in 90% of follicular-type non-Hodgkin's lymphomas [88]. This translocation places the *BCL-2*, normally located on chromosome 18, under the influence of the immunoglobulin heavy chain gene locus situated on chromosome 14 resulting in overproduction of Bcl-2 protein and prolonged survival of the malignant cells. t(14;18) was the first gene found to contribute to tumor growth by reducing cell death rather than by promoting cell division, a major breakthrough that suggests a new strategy for combating cancer. Indeed, it can be envisioned that manipulation of the pro- and anti-apoptotic forces to favor the former might in the future restore the normal apoptotic process lost during tumorigenesis, thus removing the survival advantage of malignant cells. In the interim, the near universal association of t(14;18) with follicular-type non-Hodgkin's lymphomas has diagnostic and prognostic value in the clinical setting: it serves to differentiate this relatively benign type of lymphoma from more aggressive forms of the disease and thus guide therapy.

Telomeres

At the end of each chromosome lies a unique stretch of repeated DNA sequences (TTAGGG) approximately 15,000 base pairs long, called telomeres [89]. These sequences do not contain genetic codes but are critical to the aging of normal cells and to the apparent inexhaustible ability of cancer cells to replicate. Telomeres are sometimes referred to as the cell *"clock"* or *"counting mechanism"* because they limit the number of divisions a normal cell can undertake. When a normal cell divides the ends of chromosomes cannot be replicated and 25 to 200 base pairs are lost with each division, progressively reducing the length of telomeres. Eventually, once somatic cells loose their entire telomere sequences, after multiple replication rounds, they can no longer divide and are set to die. This is because telomerase, an enzyme that restores and maintains telomere length in undifferentiated cells such as embryonic and stem cells, is repressed in normal somatic cells. In contrast, high levels of telomerase have been reported in the vast majority of human malignancies [90]. However, while telomerase activity enables malignant cells to replicate indefinitely, a property that could be exploited therapeutically, it is not involved in the development, growth, or dissemination of cancer. Telomeres and telomerase might also play a role in human aging as suggested by recent observations in experimental mice and in a rare human disease. Mice genetically modified to make them telomerase-deficient (telomerase *"knock-out"* mice) give rise to offspring whose life span is dependent on the length of their telomeres. Likewise, dyskeratosis congenita, a fatal X-linked human disease associated with decreased RNA telomerase, decreased telomerase activity, and shorter telomeres, exhibits age-dependent chromosomal abnormalities and an increased tendency to develop malignancies. Finally, while increased telomerase activity is detected in 94% of neuroblastomas, mainly a childhood cancer, low or undetectable telomerase levels are found in a disease subset called neuroblastoma 4S. Children afflicted by neuroblastoma 4S exhibit an astonishing 80% spontaneous remission rate, a behavior not seen with any other cancer. These compelling observations have lead a number of research laboratories and several biotechnology companies to actively study telomerase as a potential diagnostic and therapeutic target. For example, early-stage bladder cancer is notoriously difficult to diagnose given the absence of noticeable tumors and lack of means to differentiate cancerous from normal cells voided in the urine. Thus, a reliable test to quantify telomerase activity in urine samples could significantly improve detection of this, the 5th most frequent cancer in the US. Additionally, telomerase inhibitors with demonstrable activity in cancer cells will soon be tested in animal models, and eventually in cancer patients. It is tantalizing to contemplate the possibility that manipulation of a single molecule might one day prolong the lifespan of normal cells and by extension slow aging, and control some cancers by eliminating the survival advantage of malignant cells.

2. HOW DOES CANCER ARISE?

2.1 First the basics

A still prevailing definition of cancer calls it an "*uncontrolled cell proliferation*". While satisfactory through the 1970's, this definition is obsolete today in view of the prodigious advances made in the last 20 years regarding the genetic bases of cancer. It is now understood that exposure to noxious agents such as radiation, chemical, or viral mutagens throughout life can lead to alterations in DNA sequences. Cancer develops when 2 or more sequential DNA *"hits"* induce gene mutations that promote growth or confer a survival advantage to the affected cell and its descendents, collectively called a malignant *"clone"*. Additional critical mutations in any of these malignant clonal cells are thought necessary for a cancer to become locally or distally invasive. There are two major groups of normal cellular genes associated with cancer when mutated [91]: *Proto-oncogenes* (100 are currently known) that promote, and *tumor suppressor genes* (over 30 are known) that inhibit cell growth. Proto-oncogenes mutate (to *"oncogenes"*) via several mechanisms: amplification (multiple copies of the gene), as in the case of *Erb-B2* associated with breast cancer; point mutations (amino acid substitutions on the gene), as in the case of *RET* implicated in multiple endocrine and thyroid cancers; and gene translocation from one chromosome to another. The latter can generate a fusion (or "*chimeric*") gene, as is the case of *bcr/abl* in chronic myelogenous leukemia, or place the gene under the hyperactive control of the immunoglobulin heavy-chain locus or the T-cell receptor genes, resulting in lymphomas or leukemias. *DNA viral oncogenes* differ from cellular oncogenes in that they derive not from *cellular proto-oncogenes* but from *DNA viruses* that transcribe into infected cells the genome signals that trigger excessive cell proliferation. Perhaps the best-known example of a human DNA virus-induced cancer is cervical cancer, which is caused by several strains of the human papilloma virus. In contrast to the hyperactive growth-promoting effect of oncogenes, mutated tumor suppressor genes are deleted or loose their inhibitory function thus depriving cells of the crucial brakes that normally prevent excessive cell growth. A subset of tumor suppressor genes, called DNA repair genes were discovered studying hereditary nonpolyposis colorectal cancer. Although not directly involved in the carcinogenesis process, inactivation of these genes can lead to a defective DNA repair process and to genomic instability. In conclusion, mutated proto-oncogenes, tumor suppressor genes, and DNA repair genes become carcinogenic by promoting excessive cell growth, by failing to block the effect of oncogenes, or by enabling replication of unstable genomes, respectively. Thus, regardless of their mechanism of action, cancer cells differ from their normal counterpart in their aberrant regulation by mutated genomes, not lack thereof. The degree of deregulation determines the biology of malignant cells, which in turn dictates the clinical course of the disease, as exemplified by the two genetic variants of chronic lymphocytic leukemia [92].

The vast majority of mutations involved in cancer development affect somatic but not gonadal cells. That is, they are present only in cancer cells and are neither inherited nor inheritable. However, a small fraction of mutations are inherited, thus affecting all cells of an individual. These mutant genes predispose the host to cancer and are transmitted from generation to generation by the affected gonads. Well know examples of inherited mutant genes include *RB1*, associated with retinoblastoma of childhood, and *BRCA1* associated with familial breast cancer of young females. As mentioned earlier, cancer results from a multi-step process that over time alters one or more genes. Thus, the chances that a single cell (out of 10^{14} that make up a human being) would undergo several successive mutations is negligible, were it not for the fact that some mutations affect the stability of the genome, increasing its susceptibility to additional damage. In the case of somatic mutations, genetic damage occurs over many years, which accounts for the advanced age of the vast majority of cancer patients. In contrast, in individuals born with a cancer-predisposing gene all cells are already mutated, thus vastly expanding the cell pool susceptible to additional mutations, increasing the cancer risk, and the likelihood that the disease will appear in childhood or early adulthood.

Oncogenes, tumor suppressor genes, and DNA repair genes are described in greater detail in the following pages. Readers not particularly interested in such details can proceed to the segment *How does cancer spread?*, starting on page 58.

2.2 More details

Oncogenes and Proto-oncogenes. Oncogenes were discovered through the study of retroviruses, which are RNA tumor viruses. The oncogene-containing genome of retroviruses is inserted into the DNA of infected cells, a process called *"insertional mutagenesis"*. This causes malignant transformation of the infected cell(s) and production of viral progeny that by infecting other cells perpetuate the process. Studies of Rous sarcoma virus (RSV) mutants revealed that the transforming gene (*v-src*) of this retrovirus was not necessary for viral replication, and that it had a counterpart gene (*c-src*) in normal cells. This surprising discovery, confirmed in all retroviruses studied, demonstrated that retroviral oncogenes (*v-onc*) are altered versions of normal cellular proto-oncogenes. In rare cases, weak oncogenic retroviruses initiate a mutagenic event that activates cellular proto-oncogenes. Many proto-oncogenes, also called "*accelerator*" genes, encode growth-promoting proteins that relay growth signals from outside the cell through a cascade pathway that begins at the level of cell membrane receptors and ends in the cell nucleus. The sequence is as follows: growth-promoting proteins attach to the extra-cellular portion of specific receptors on target cells. Attachment triggers a stimulatory signal down the intra-cellular portion of the receptor reaching the cell nucleus through a series of complex pathways referred to as the "*signal transduction cascade*". In the nucleus, another set of proteins called "*transcription factors*" steer the cell through its replication cycle (cell cycle). Each growth-promoting step is associated with proto-oncogenes, resulting in five classes of such genes: growth factors or external signals, growth factor receptors, signal transducers, transcription factors, and regulators of the cell cycle. Given the complexity and heterogeneity of cancer, it was predicted that each class of proto-oncogenes would have a corresponding oncogene. Indeed, such is the case. An example of growth factor oncogene is seen in dermatofibrosarcoma protuberans, a form of human skin cancer, where a fusion gene gives rise to excessive amounts of platelet-dependent growth factor-beta (*PDGF-β*), a growth signal that auto-stimulates the PDGF-receptor bearing cancer cells that produce it. Other growth factors include nerve growth factor, epidermal growth factor, and fibroblast growth factor. Likewise, oncogenic receptor genes have been identified. These mutated genes encode production of abnormal receptors, such as e*rb-B2* in breast cancer, that spontaneously fire proliferative signals down the intra-cellular cascade without the stimulus of extracellular growth factors. Signal transducer oncogenes include the prominent *ras* family, which is active in approximately 25% of colon, lung, and pancreas cancers. While the normal *ras* proto-oncogene mediates normal growth receptor signals downstream, the mutated *ras* oncogene fires continuously and independently of any receptor gene signal, pushing cancer growth forward. Transcriptional oncogenes, such as the *myc* family, are amplified in 20% to 30% of all cancers, including squamous cell carcinomas, neuroblastoma, and lung cancer, but are crucial to the development of all Burkitt's lymphoma. This aggressive lymphoma is characterized by translocation of the *c-myc* normally located at 8q24 (band 24 of the long arm of chromosome 8), to 14q32 (band 32 of the long arm of chromosome 14) where it falls under the control of the immunoglobulin heavy-chain locus, leading to enhanced proliferation of malignant cells.

Tumor suppressor genes (Table VI). An entirely different class of genes, known as tumor suppressor or "*brake*" genes, ensures that normal cells possess effective breaks to balance the effect of growth promoting proteins.

Like oncogenes, tumor suppressor genes contribute to cancer development through structural or functional alterations that range from point mutations to deletions of the entire chromosome where they reside. However, unlike oncogenes that are activated versions of proto-oncogenes, mutated suppressor genes are inactivated or deleted versions of their normal counterparts that lead to *"loss of function"* when both alleles (inherited one per parent) are involved. Loss of function promotes cancer development through several mechanisms but mainly via releasing cells from normal proliferative breaks, or by reinforcing the over-stimulatory effect of oncogenes. Retinoblastoma and breast cancer best illustrate these most clinically relevant genes. Retinoblastoma is a rare but aggressive childhood cancer of the retina caused by inactivated *RB1,* which is located at 13q14 (region 14 of long arm of chromosome 13). Approximately 60% of retinoblastomas are sporadic that occur in individuals with no family history of the disease, and are always unilateral. The other 40% are inherited and are frequently bilateral. In sporadic cases, both *RB1* alleles are functional in normal cells but inactive in tumor cells. In contrast, only one *RB1* allele is functional in normal cells of inherited cases. Thus, while in sporadic cases two consecutive mutations are required to inactivate the two previously normal *RB1* alleles, individuals born with only one functional *RB1* allele will develop retinoblastoma after a single mutation, and will do so at an earlier age. In fact, 80% of inherited retinoblastomas are diagnosed before age 3. Breast cancer is usually a sporadic malignancy. However, approximately 20% of cases occur at an earlier age, in families that inherit germline mutations of *BRCA1* and less frequently *BRCA2.* Mutations of *BRCA1,* located at 17q21 (region 21 of long arm of chromosome 17) and *BRCA2,* located at 13q12-13 (bands 12-13 of long arm of chromosome 13), are associated with an increased risk of breast cancer and an earlier onset. *BRCA1* exhibits an approximately 85% life-long risk of female breast cancer. *BRCA2* is associated with a 40% and 10% risk of female breast and ovarian cancer, respectively, and accounts for approximately 5% of male breast cancer cases. Finally, recent evidence suggests that a third tumor-suppressor, breast cancer-associated gene *(BRCA3),* also located on chromosome 13, might account for familial cases lacking *BRCA1* and *BRCA2.*

DNA repair genes. A distinct subclass of tumor suppressor genes is engaged in DNA damage recognition and repair. In contrast to dominant tumor suppressor genes (such as *RB1* and *TP53*) that actively promote cancer development, mutated DNA repair genes exert a more passive role in carcinogenesis: they fail to detect and repair DNA damage during the cell cycle.

Table VI. Tumor-suppressor genes (partial list). Reproduced (with modifications) with permission from Nat Med 10:409:850-852, 2001

Gene (synonym(s))	Syndrome	Cancer type
APC	Familial polyposis of colon	Colon, Thyroid, Gastrointestinal
AXIN2	Attenuated polyposis	Colon
BMPR1A	Juvenile polyposis	Gastrointestinal
BRCA1, BRCA2	Hereditary breast cancer	Familial Breast/Ovarian
BHD	Birt-Hogg-Dube	Renal
CDH1 (E-cadherin)	Familial gastric carcinoma	Stomach
CDK4	Familial malignant melanoma	Melanoma
CDKN2A(p16^{INK4A}, p14^{ARF})	Familial malignant melanoma	Melanoma, Pancreas
CYLD	Familial cylindromatosis	Pilotricomas
EXT1,2	Hereditary multiple exostoses	Osteosarcoma
FH	Hereditary leiomyomatosis	Leiomyomas
GPC3	Simpson-Golabi-Behmel	Embryonal
HRPT2	Hyperparathyroidism Jaw-tumor	Parathyroid, Jaw fibromas
MEN1	Multiple endocrine neoplasia	Parathyroid, Pituitary, Islet cell
NF2	Neurofibromatosis type 2	Meningioma, Acoustic neuroma
PTEN	Cowden	Hamartoma, Glioma, Endometrial
PTCH	Gorlin	Basal cell, Medulloblastoma
RB1	Hereditary retinoblastoma	Retinoblastoma & Others
SDHB, C, D	Familial paraganglioma	Paragangliomas,
SMAD4 (DPC4)	Juvenile polyposis	Gastrointestinal
SUFU	Medulloblastoma predisposition	Skin, Medulloblastoma
STK11 (LKB1)	Peutz-Jeghers	Intestinal, Ovarian, Pancreatic
TP53 (p53)	Li-Fraumeni	Breast, Sarcoma, Adrenal, Brain
TSC1, TSC2	Tuberous sclerosis	Hamartoma, Reanl
VHL	Von Hippel–Lindau	Renal
WT1	Familial Wilms tumor	Wilms'

Most errors in DNA sequence prevent cell replication or are lethal to the cell. However, a few unrepaired DNA errors will enter the cell cycle thus increasing the frequency of random tumor-promoting mutations in daughter cells and the risk of cancer. Examples of inherited cancer predisposition resulting from a defective DNA damage recognition and repair system include Ataxia-Telangiectasia, Bloom syndrome, Xeroderma pigmentosa, Fanconi's anemia, and Hereditary nonpolyposis colorectal cancer. However, only homozygotes (individuals who inherit a mutated allele from each parent) appear to have a clear cancer predisposition, in contrast to the more dominant tumor suppressor genes *RB1* and *TP53* that increase cancer risk in heterozygous individuals (individuals with only one mutated allele).

3.   HOW DOES CANCER SPREAD?

Normal cells discharge their multiple functions within the anatomical confines of the organ they constitute. For example, normal liver cells remain within the liver and are never found in brains, kidneys, lungs, or elsewhere. Even blood cells that circulate throughout the body to deliver oxygen, to seek and kill invading bacteria, and to plug vascular leaks do not disrupt the function of the tissues they serve. Benign tumors, on the other hand, have a tendency to expand concentrically causing compression of contiguous tissues without invading local or distant sites. Except when located in vital organs such as brain and heart, benign tumors normally constitute no threat to the host despite occasionally reaching enormous sizes, as can occur in geographic areas with primitive health care. In contrast, cancer cells possess the inherent ability to trespass into the spaces of adjacent and distant tissues. The ability of cancer to aberrantly invade contiguous tissues and to spread (*"metastasize"*) to distant sites is the hallmark of malignancy. By destroying or compromising the structure or the function of invaded normal tissues, metastases are life-threatening to the host. Patients' outcomes are ultimately dependent upon the invasiveness and metastatic potential of their cancer. Indeed, early stage malignancies not accompanied by distant metastases are curable by surgical extirpation. However, approximately 30% of cancer patients have disseminated disease or detectable metastases at the time of diagnosis, and another 20% to 30% have occult metastases or will develop them later, as revealed by their subsequent clinical course. Hence, a single metastasis regardless of size is an indication of widespread disease no longer amenable to cure, particularly given their frequently inaccessible anatomic location in lungs, liver, brain, and bones, and the limited efficacy of chemotherapy and radiation therapy.

3.1   Local invasiveness

Cancer invasiveness and the potential to metastasize are related but distinct processes under different genetic control. Each process requires a series of sequential steps, called the invasiveness and metastatic cascades, that represent aberrations of the normal processes that keep normal cells in place within their designated spaces. Normal cells adhere to one another through cell-adhesion molecules such as *E-cadherins*. E-cadherins also play a role in the ability of malignant cells to form tumors and invade tissues [93]. For example, blocking E-cadherins can turn stationary cells into invasive ones. Alternatively, restoring E-cadherins in cancer cells deprived of this molecule prevents these cells from forming tumors. On the other hand, cell adherence to the extra cellular matrix, a process mediated by *integrins*, enables cells to survive and proliferate. Without matrix anchorage, normal cells cannot survive and undergo apoptosis. There is experimental evidence suggesting that anchorage is tissue-specific; that is, a detached normal cell cannot anchor itself in a tissue other that its own. In contrast, helped by molecules such as cyclin E-CDK2 cancer cells can survive for long periods without matrix anchorage or adhere to matrixes of unrelated tissues, conferring these cells the potential to form metastases.

3.2   Metastases

In order to metastasize cancer cells must detach from their original anchorage site, invade a blood vessel or lymphatic channel, travel passively to a distant site, establish a new tumor colony, and trigger new blood vessel formation. As they travel, cancer cells eventually become trapped in the smallest blood vessels (capillaries) or in lymph nodes that, interspersed in the lymphatic system, act as temporary barriers. However, not all cancer cells that migrate from the primary site will establish a distant colony. Indeed, the hurdles to a cancer cell in the metastatic cascade are multiple and the process is highly inefficient as shown by the rarity of metastases given the millions of cancer cells shed by a cancer into the circulation each day [94]. Evaluation of the extent (or "*stage*") of disease, especially a search for metastases, is crucial to patient management as it provides the basis for treatment decisions and for assessing prognosis. For example, breast cancer surgery includes assessment of the status of axillary lymph nodes draining the affected breast: negative lymph nodes suggest a cancer restricted to the breast and a favorable prognosis. Alternatively, cancer-positive nodes indicate that cancer cells have migrated outside the breast and have likely metastasized to distant sites, auguring a poor prognosis. Indeed, the presence of metastases plays a pivotal role on patient survival regardless of the origin and type of cancer. For example, approximately 90% of patients with colon cancer restricted to the gut wall live 5 years after diagnosis, whereas only 65% will live 5 years after cancer cells have invaded regional lymph nodes [95]. Likewise, 90% of women with localized breast cancer survive 10 years, but only 15% do so if distant metastases are present [95]. *In vitro* and *in vivo* animal studies conducted in the last decade have demonstrated the existence of human metastasis-promoting genes (WDNM-1, WDNM-2, MMP11, MTA1 and ERBB2), and metastasis-suppressor genes (nm23, KAI1, KiSS1, BrMS1 and MKK4 [96]). While these data are derived from animal studies, their potential application in the clinical setting cannot be underestimated. For example, a decreased expression of nm23 and/or E-cadherin combined with high blood vessel count in the primary tumors of breast cancer patients might be a better indicator of poor prognosis than an advanced tumor stage

[97,98]. Thus, one of the challenges for the future is to identify genetic profiles underlying metastatic potential.

PART III

HOW IS CANCER TREATED?

Chapter 5

THE CANCER CELL-KILL PARADIGM AND ITS COROLLARIES

Implicit in the term neoplasm or *"new growth"* is the notion that cancer, like invading bacteria, is inherently different from the host and must be thoroughly eradicated in order to prevent recurrences and death. The application of the infectious disease model to cancer steered cancer research, diagnosis, treatment, and outcome assessment strategies towards the cancer cell-killing paradigm. That is, like invading bacteria, cancer must be eradicated before it overwhelms the host. From this basis, two major practical corollaries followed. The first is that cancer research has been oriented towards the search for therapeutically exploitable differences between cancer and normal cells, guided by successive hypotheses ranging from excessive cancer cell proliferation [1], a misconceived generalization that drove drug use for decades, to tumor-specific antigens targetable for therapy [2]; an illusion not yet abandoned. As decried in a recent article [3], *"medical treatment of cancer for most of the past century was like trying to fix an automobile without any knowledge of the internal combustion engines or, for that matter, even the ability to look under the hood"*. The second corollary is the concept of *"cytotoxicity"* (or cell killing) that was introduced to describe the quintessential property that drugs must exhibit in order to be successful in the treatment of disseminated cancer. However, how were these drugs to preferentially kill cancer cells while sparing normal cells was never adequately explored nor fully explained. The notion of cell-killing as the cornerstone of cancer treatment became untenable when the carcinogenic process was shown to involve oncogenes that promote cell growth, mutated tumor suppressor genes that fail to counteract cancer-promoting oncogenes, defective DNA repair genes that enable replication and propagation of unstable genomes, or faulty cell death pathways that confer a survival advantage to cancer cells.

From this flawed concept about cancer treatment an entire lexicon was developed in attempts to explain empirical clinical observations. For example, the tendency of some tumors to outgrow adjacent normal tissues, a phenomenon that can be slowed and sometimes reverted by anti-cancer drugs, suggested a pivotal role for the cell cycle in tumor growth and anti-cancer drug activity. Thus, cancer drugs were classified as *"cell cycle dependent"* if they acted upon one of the phases of the cell cycle, and *"cell cycle independent"* if their anti-tumor activity was independent of the cell cycle. The former in turn were classified as S-specific (drugs that inhibit DNA synthesis, such as the antimetabolites and antipurines), M-phase dependent (drugs that arrest mitosis, such as Vinca alkaloids, Podophyllotoxins and Taxanes), or G_1- and G_2-phase dependent, such as Corticosteroids and Asparaginase, and Bleomycin and Topotecan, respectively. Cell-cycle independent drugs included all the alkylators, such as Busulfan, Melphalan, and Chlorambucil. Mechanism of action to a large degree determined the type of toxicity. Likewise, it was quickly discovered that anti-tumor activity was dose-dependent and that dose escalation was limited by type and level of toxicity resulting from drug effect on normal cells. Thus, in order to enhance anti-tumor activity with tolerable toxicity, drugs with different mechanisms of action and toxicities were combined and administered intermittently, enabling normal tissues, especially the bone marrow, to recover between treatment cycles. Perhaps the most successful example of this approach was the MOPP (Nitrogen mustard, Vincristine, Prednisone, and Procarbazine) chemotherapy regimen for Hodgkin's disease that proved curative in most cases [4]. However, this early success was seldom replicated despite a myriad of subsequent clinical trials launched to test a variety of intermittent combination chemotherapy regimens in many types of cancers over the ensuing four decades.

In response to the marginal results achieved by cytotoxic chemotherapy in the management of most advanced malignancies, cancer researchers explored new treatment modalities with renewed enthusiasm and unrealistic expectations. One such direction was based on the *"immune surveillance"* hypothesis that emerged from observations made in the 1960s of an increased cancer risk in patients with severe congenital or acquired immunodeficiencies [5]. According to this hypothesis, cancer cells emerge from time to time but are eliminated by a sort of search-and-destroy defense mechanism before they can develop into full-blown tumors. Defects in *immune surveillance* were believed not only to contribute to cancer development but also to prevent the elimination of a few cancer cells remaining after successful chemotherapy, thus leading to relapses. This conceptually attractive hypothesis found widespread following. For example, at the *International Conference on Immune Surveillance* held at Brook Lodge, MI in May 1970 [6], the Chairman opened the meeting declaring, *"Everyone here surely accepts the reality of tumor-specific immunity and would also favor the proposition that cell-mediated immune mechanisms have something to do with recognition and attack on tumor-specific antigens"*. It was proposed that immune defects could be overcome by immune stimulants. Experimental attempts to potentiate the cancer-fighting capacity of the immune system began in the mid-1960s for the treatment of childhood leukemia [7], using BCG (Bacillus Calmette Guérin), a laboratory bacterium derived from Mycobacterium Tuberculosis. The Interferons [8], Levamisole [9], and the more toxic Interleukins [10] followed this in the 1970s and 1980s. As the concept of cancer immunotherapy gathered momentum, new agents were grouped under the evocative name *"Biological Response Modifiers"*. Their mechanism of action was thought to *"alter the interactions between the body's immune defenses and cancer to boost, direct, or restore the body's ability to fight the disease"*. Each immune enhancer rode a wave of enthusiasm within the medical community and in the press. For example, Interferon was greeted with a deluge of media coverage thanks to astute promoters. It was touted a *"magic bullet"*, a *"miracle cure"*, *"Like the genie in a fairy tale"* that was equally good to cure the common cold or cancer. Business journalists touted Interferon as a *"gold mine for patients and for companies"*, and as a result stock prices of manufacturing firms rose dramatically. In the late 1970s, the American Cancer Society awarded a 2-million dollar grant, the largest in its history, to conduct clinical trials. In May 1980, based on unpublished clinical trial results, a the *New York Times* article raised doubts about the anti-cancer efficacy of Interferon. In response to the article, four scientists from the Sloan Kettering Institute for Cancer Research wrote a letter to the newspaper expressing dismay that such reporting might undermine public support of interferon research. Eventually, as discouraging results of clinical trials became known, the public mood switched from premature enthusiasm to pessimism, especially when four patients treated with interferon in France died as result of the treatment. Using interferon as an example, an analysis [11] of historical medical news reporting by the media made the following observations on its impact on science, *"First, imagery often replaced content"*. *"Second, the press covered interferon research as a series of dramatic events. Readers were treated to hyperbole, to promotional coverage designed to raise their expectations and whet their interest."* The role of scientists was described as follows, *"Far from being neutral sources of information, scientists themselves actively sought a favorable press, equating public interest with research support."* Interleukin-2 was another darling of the media through the 1990s, as typified by the numerous guest appearances of its main promoter in ABC's *"World News Tonight with Peter Jennings"*.

Despite two decades of intense studies, immune stimulants have had little impact on cancer management. BCG is used successfully for treating the relatively few cases of *in situ* bladder cancer. Interferons are very active in Hairy cell leukemia, an extremely rare form of the leukemia (fewer than 700 yearly cases in the US), and are marginally beneficial to 15% of patients with disseminated skin melanoma and kidney cancer. Likewise, interleukin-2 is marginally effective in approximately 15% of patients with skin melanoma, kidney cancer, and non-Hodgkin's lymphoma [12], despite its high toxicity. Ignoring reality, its main proponent recently concluded [12], *"The demonstration that even bulky invasive tumours can undergo complete regression under appropriate immune stimulation by IL-2 has shown that it is indeed possible to treat cancer successfully by immune manipulation"*. Thus, after years of clinical trials, at great human and financial cost, immune stimulants have shown marginal usefulness in cancer management despite their moderate to marked toxicity. A variant of immunotherapy use putative tumor antigens [12] as targets for drug development or for generating immune-enhancing vaccines. In the last ten years, a number of clinical trials were designed to assess the efficacy of various vaccine strategies to induce antigen-specific immune responses in cancer patients. Strategies ranged from whole cancer cells or cancer cell-derived single-antigen peptides, used alone or as complex cocktails of antigen peptides, in combination with cytokines or adjuvants (agents that enhance the presumed immunogenecity of antigens) [13]. However, it now appears clear that most cancers develop, not as a result of immune deficiencies or by escaping immune detection but precisely because cancer cells do not exhibit any distinct feature recognizable by the host's immune system. Not surprisingly, only occasional immunity-related tumor responses have been observed, and they have occurred independently of the vaccination strategy or immunotherapy maneuvers, suggesting that manipulation of the immune system is unlikely to find a prominent role in future cancer management.

Another direction of the *War on Cancer* that generated enormous enthusiasm and consumed large resources was the virus link. The old hypothesis that viruses were responsible for most cancers was revived with renewed interest following the discovery of the first retrovirus in 1981 [14], and of the HIV two years later [15]. This new direction in cancer research, vigorously promoted and generously funded by NCI, helped establish or confirm a cancer link to several viruses, including HTLV-1 retroviruses (T-cell lymphomas) [15], Herpes viruses (cavitary lymphomas) [16], Papilloma virus (cervical cancer) [17], certain adenoviruses (liver cancer) [18,19], and Epstein-Barr virus (Burkitt's lymphoma and pharyngeal cancer) [20]. It also led to major advances in molecular biology especially in AIDS. However, by the mid 1980s it became clear that the notion that most cancers were caused by viruses was a false lead and the idea was discarded. Nevertheless, prophylactic vaccination of populations at risk of exposure to cancer-promoting viruses is likely to play a significant role in future cancer prevention, as discussed in chapter 12. Neither the immune or viral links to cancer, nor attempts to optimize the efficacy of cytotoxic chemotherapy through dose escalation and drug combinations yielded the anticipated therapeutic success. Today, while nearly 50% of resectable cancers are cured by surgery, fewer than 2% of patients with advanced or metastatic cancers will experience a sustained disease-free survival, demonstrating the superiority of prevention and early-stage diagnosis over treating advanced disease with drugs. More on this in Chapters 7 and 12.

Early-stage diagnosis has been facilitated by technological advances in imaging and molecular tools that have propelled cancer diagnosis from the clinical to the molecular realm. These include: 1) imaging techniques such as computerized axial tomography (CAT-scan), magnetic resonance imaging (MRI), and ultrasound all suited to detect cancer at the multi-cellular level; 2) cellular and molecular methods such as cytogenetics (including fluorescence in-situ hybridization, comparative genomic hybridization, spectral karyotype, and microarray techniques), flow cytometry, and polymerase chain reaction (PCR) capable of detecting abnormalities at the subcellular or molecular levels [21,22]; and 3) routine laboratory testing for cancer cell products, such as serum levels of monoclonal immunoglobulins, PSA and CEA associated with multiple myeloma, prostate, and colon cancer, respectively. For example, PCR, a powerful molecular tool applicable to hematologic malignancies, enables detection of as few as one leukemia or lymphoma cell out of 1 million normal cells [22]. Such remarkable discriminant diagnostic power has thrusted the definition and notion of complete remission from the clinical and pathologic domains to the molecular realm. This new goal has had the unintended consequence of fostering more aggressive and prolonged chemotherapy in attempts to eradicate the very last detectable cancer cell, inevitably resulting in greater toxicity. However, regardless of its definition, complete remissions are rarely achieved and true cures remain elusive, forcing the coinage of an entire lexicon of terms designed to characterize and quantify intermediate treatment outcomes. These fall under two general categories: tumor outcomes ranging from a lack of response to a complete remission, and patient outcomes, most importantly prolongation of survival and quality of life. Tumor outcome assessment is useful as an early indication of the effectiveness of a particular therapy but not to predict survival, although prolongation of survival is generally preceded by complete remissions. On the other hand, patient outcome assessment constitutes the ultimate standard to gauge the success or failure of patient management, as advocated by the Health Services Research Committee of the American Society of Clinical Oncology [23]. However, because patient outcome is judged in retrospect and tumor response is immediate, in the practice setting tumor responses are interpreted as the first step towards a complete remission and, it is hoped, prolonged survival. The fallacy of this approach is that while most patients achieve some degree of tumor response few survive longer as a result. Survival rates are said to be *relative* when they represent the survival rates a group of cancer patients compared to the survival rates for persons in the general population matched for age, gender, race, and calendar year of observation. Relative survival also adjusts for life expectancy in the population at large. Unless qualified (such as disease-free or relapse-free), relative survival rates include persons who are living after diagnosis, whether or not disease-free, often times reflecting factors unrelated to the particular cancer or its treatment. While all these terms were designed to compare and communicate outcomes of clinical cancer research, tumor response has been adopted in the clinical setting as an indication of treatment success or failure because its immediacy is attractive to physicians and patients despite not predicting survival. Unfortunately, focusing on tumor responses rather than on patient survival, an implicit acknowledgment of the unresponsiveness of most cancers, detracts clinicians from their primary purpose, mainly designing a management plan to optimize patient welfare rather than to maximize tumor shrinkage at any cost. This practice also misleads patients given the promises implied in words such a *"response"* and *"remission"*, as discussed in chapter 11.

Chapter 6

CHEMOTHERAPY DRUGS

1.   HISTORICAL BACKGROUND: MUSTARD GAS

While surgery is most adept and successful at managing early stage cancer, Medical Oncology is the discipline that uses drugs for treating advanced, inoperable cancer. Today, the vast majority of patients with disseminated or metastatic cancer are treated with drugs either alone or in combination with surgery or radiotherapy. As briefly reviewed in chapter 3, herbs, potions, and topical agents have been used to treat cancer for many centuries. However, systemic cancer chemotherapy is a recent development with its historical origins in observations of the toxic effects on humans accidentally exposed to chemical warfare agents, mainly mustard gas, during WWI and WWII, and to experimental studies of these agents used systemically in animals and humans preceding and during WWII. Mustard gas is the common name for 1,1-thiobis(2-chloroethane), a vesicant chemical warfare agent synthesized by Frederick Guthrie in 1860 and first used near Ypres (Belgium) during WWI. Thus, its alternate name, Yperite. Because it could penetrate masks and other protective materials available during WWI, and given its widespread use by both sides of the conflict, its effects were particularly horrific and deadly. Out of 1,205,655 individuals exposed to Mustard gas during WWI, 91,198 died [24]. It was at this time that mustard gas victims were first noted to develop low white blood cell counts and bone marrow aplasia. In a landmark study [25], a group of researchers at the University of Pennsylvania conducted autopsies on 75 soldiers who died of exposure to mustard gas during WWI, and reported decreased white blood cell counts and depletion of the bone marrow and lymphoid tissues. Shortly

69

thereafter, military researchers from the US Chemical Warfare Service reported the same effects in rabbits injected intravenously with dichloroethylsulfide contaminated with mustard gas [26]. Fifteen years later the anti-cancer activity of mustard gas in experimental animal models was reported for the first time [27]. During WWII, the US's Office of Scientific Research and Development (OSRD) funded Yale University to conduct, in secrecy, chemical welfare research [28]. These studies lead to the confirmation of the anti-tumor activity of mustard gas in murine lymphoma, and to the first human trials of nitrogen mustard reported at a Chicago meeting in early 1943 [29]. However, what brought the medical community's attention to the Yale's group studies and launched the era of cancer chemotherapy was a WWII incident when humans were accidentally exposed to mustard gas released during the bombardment of the Italian town of Bari by Hitler's Luftwaffe, on December 2, 1943.

Bari was a usually sleepy town of approximately 65,000 people located on the Adriatic shore of the Italian "*boot*". Old Bari, perched on a promontory around its medieval fortified Castello Normanno Svevo and the Basilica San Nicolo, and new Bari, were transformed in late 1943 by the arrival of approximately 30 allied ships in its small harbor. Under British jurisdiction, Bari was the main supply center for British General Montgomery's Army, and had just been designated headquarters of the American Fifteenth Air Force division. Occasionally, German reconnaissance planes would fly over Bari undisturbed by the Allies who believed that the Luftwaffe was spread too thin to mount a successful attack on the city. In the early afternoon of December 2, 1943 Werner Hahn flying his Messerschmitt Me-210 reconnaissance plane made two undisturbed high altitude passes over the city, reporting to his superiors the suitability of Bari as a target for an air strike. Later that day, British Air Vice-Marshall Sir Arthur Conningham held a press conference. Answering war correspondents' pointed questions regarding lax security he declared, with characteristic British self-confidence, "*I would consider it a personal insult if the enemy should send so much as one plane over the city*". A few hours later a squadron of 105 twin-engine Junkers Ju-88 A-4 bombers lead by Lieutenant Gustav Teuber left their base in northern Italy and, flying low to evade Allied radar, descended on Bari in a surprise air strike that would become known as "*the second Pearl Harbor*". When the squadron arrived, the German pilots could hardly believe their eyes and their luck: The entire harbor was brightly lit highlighting ships and personnel unloading cargo! At 7:50 PM, twenty minutes after the raid began, eight allied ships had been damaged and fifteen were sunk, including the John Harvey, an American ship, with its secret load of 100 tons of Mustard gas. A few rounds fired by the sole, antiquated anti-aircraft battery in the city had been futile. After the explosions, fire was everywhere. Flames engulfed damaged and sinking ships, as well as patches of oil and debris floating on the water. At first, casualties seemed relatively modest given the extent of materiel losses. However, many survivors exhibited severe eye irritation, skin rashes, and other symptoms not usually seen among war casualties and doctors began suspecting that the Luftwaffe had used chemical warfare. Informed of the mysterious malady, Deputy Surgeon General Fred Blesse dispatched Lt. Col. Stewart Francis Alexander, an American physician expert in chemical warfare. From his clinical and pathologic studies, Dr. Alexander suspected mustard gas. Carefully tallying the location of the victims at the time of the attack, he was able to trace the epicenter to the John Harvey, confirming mustard gas as the culprit when he located a fragment of an American M47A1 bomb, he knew carried the agent. This would be the only episode of exposure to a chemical warfare agent during WWII. By the end of the month, 83 of the 628 hospitalized military mustard gas victims had died. The number of civilian casualties, thought to have been even greater, could not be ascertained accurately because most had sought refuge with relatives out of town. Allied Supreme Commander General Dwight D. Eisenhower approved Dr. Alexander's full report [30]. British Primer Minister Winston S. Churchill ordered all British documents to be purged, listing mustard gas deaths as *"burns due to enemy action"*.

2. FIFTY YEARS OF ANTI-CANCER DRUG DISCOVERY: THE ROLE OF SERENDIPITY AND TRIAL & ERROR

The notion that the suppressive effect of mustard gas on bone marrow and lymphoid tissues could be exploited for therapeutic gain was not suggested until 1935 [27]. Moreover, it would take another fifteen years when the converging impacts of the 1943 Bari incident and of the Yale group's work in humans prompted an intense search for agents active against cancer cells but harmless to normal cells. Of the thousands of compounds produced and hundreds tested in animal models, Nitrogen Mustard (a substance where the sulfur atom on the Mustard gas is substituted by a nitrogen atom) emerged as the first agent with anti-cancer activity similar to its parent compound but with less toxicity. Lifting of the US OSRD publication ban in 1946 resulted in a series of clinical trial reports demonstrating the therapeutic effect of mustard agents in a variety of human malignancies [31-34], ushering the birth of modern cancer chemotherapy. Numerous mustard derivatives were synthesized, producing agents with anti-cancer activity including some still in use today, such as Myleran, Chlorambucil, and

Melphalan. However, initial enthusiasm was tempered by the transient nature of tumor responses and the inescapable relapses. It would take twenty-five years of trial and error to discover the optimal utilization of nitrogen mustard that combined with other drugs is capable of inducing long-term, disease-free survival in most patients with advanced Hodgkin's disease [4]. In the meantime, recognition of the role of p-aminobenzoic acid in the anti-streptococcal activity of sulfa drugs [35] lead to a rational proposal for a new direction in drug development [36]. This resulted in the synthesis of anti-folic acid antagonists Aminopterin [37] and Amethopterin (today's Methotrexate) [38]. The latter was responsible for the first temporary remissions in acute childhood leukemia, in 1948, [39] and the first cure of widespread cancer (gestational choriocarcinoma) a few years later [40]. These successes stimulated the synthesis of numerous purines and pyrimidines antagonists, including 6-mercaptopurine [41] and thioguanine [42], both still in use today. However, serendipity played a pivotal role in the discovery of numerous cancer drugs, including vinca alkaloids, epipodophyllotoxins, and platinum. Indeed, the approach to cancer drug development via mass screening of thousands of natural and synthetic compounds, a process pioneered by Paul Ehrlich at the turn of the 20th century in his 7-year quest to find anti-microbial agents, had begun.

The drug screening approach can be traced back to the prevailing tenet as the National Cancer Act of 1971 was being debated. Sidney Farber, its main proponent, declared before a House Health Subcommittee hearing, *"it is not necessary for us to make great progress in the cure of cancer, for us to have the full solution of all the problems of basic research"* (because) *"the history of Medicine is replete with examples of cures obtained years, decades and even centuries before the mechanism of action was understood for these cures"* [43]. Three decades later, the process of anti-cancer drug development remains mostly anchored on this century-old, conceptually antiquated, technically inefficient, labor intensive, costly, and low-yield "*hit-and-miss*" (mostly miss) screening approach engineered and sponsored by the National Cancer Institute (NCI). Indeed, in a massive, highly complex, and far-reaching undertaking, the NCI's Developmental Therapeutics Program has operated a repository of natural and synthetic products that have been evaluated as potential anticancer agents over the last 30 years. The repository, run by a private contractor, has accumulated over 600,000 compounds gathered from the world over. Additionally, since 1986 over 50,000 samples of plants and over 10,000 samples of marine invertebrates and algae from tropical and subtropical waters were added to the repository. The potential anti-cancer activity of each sample is assessed according to its capacity to inhibit the growth of 60 cancer cell-lines (known as NCI-60) as part of NCI's "*In vitro Cell Line Screening Project*". This project, fully implemented in 1990, has screened approximately 2,500 compounds per year using sequential steps, as follows [44]: New compounds are first pre-screened for *in vitro* activity against 3 human cancer cell lines. If the growth of at least one cell line is inhibited, the compound is tested against each of the cell lines included in NCI-60. If one or more cell lines are killed, or its growth is inhibited at very low concentrations, or it has a unique mechanism of action, the compound progresses to the next step. At this point, the compound is tested against a standard panel of 12 tumor cell lines placed in individual *"hollow-fibers"* (small tubes that retain cells but are permeable to the compounds tested) and implanted in mice. Implanted mice are then administered the compound at two different doses and 4 days later the hollow-fibers are retrieved and analyzed for cell density. Agents that retard cell growth in implanted hollow-fibers are tested in mice transplanted with specific human cancers. Compounds that inhibit tumor growth after approximately 30 days with minimal animal toxicity become eligible for pharmacology and toxicology studies in animal models and in humans and, if successful, become eligible for clinical trials (described in the section *Clinical trials* in Chapter 8).

NCI's drug development program was expected to expose growth inhibition patterns that would uncover groups of agents with distinct mechanisms of actions that in turn might reveal their molecular targets. However, no existing laboratory method can accurately predict the anti-cancer efficacy of a particular chemical and, despite high hopes and years of labor-intensive and costly search, relatively few clinically useful new cancer drugs emerged from NCI's Developmental Therapeutics Program. Indeed, according to recent NCI data [44], of 70,702 compounds screened between 1990 and 1998, 6,452 showed potential *in vitro* activity, 1,546 were chosen for testing in mice, 79 revealed some activity against human tumor cells, of which 10 (or 1.4 per 10,000 screened agents) were eligible for toxicity trials in animals and humans. Drugs that can be partly traced to this trial-and-error drug discovery process include Paclitaxel, Fludarabine, BCNU, Carboplatin, DTIC, Cytosine arabinoside, Pentostatin, Hydroxyurea, Mitoxantrone, and Topotecan, though NCI claims *"Half of the FDA-approved anticancer drugs were sponsored by NCI"* [44]. Cytosine arabinoside, inspired by C-nucleoside derived compounds isolated from the Caribbean sponge *Cryototheca crypta*, and its fluorinated derivative Gemcitabine are the only cancer drugs rising from the sea. This drug development strategy gives additional meaning to the view, expressed at the turn of the century, that *"The fields and forests, the apothecary shop and temple have been ransacked for some successful means of relief from this intractable malady. Hardly any animal has escaped making its contribution in hide or hair, tooth or toenail, thymus or thyroid, liver or spleen, in the vain search for means of relief"* [45]. Yet, all drugs generated by this discovery process are cancer non-specific, cytotoxic agents exhibiting a narrow "*therapeutic window*" (the margin between therapeutic and toxic effects) that renders them largely inefficacious against cancer but toxic to normal cells. Attempts to enhance anti-cancer activity while minimizing toxicity have achieved neither, as described below.

3.   FORTY YEARS OF ATTEMPTS TO OVERCOME CANCER DRUG INEFFICACY

As of this writing (updated in May 2004) there are 76 distinct FDA-approved anti-cancer (also called anti-neoplastic or cytotoxic) drugs at our disposal (Figure 13). Seventeen of these were classified by a recent report from the WHO [46] as "*essential*" for the treatment of "*curable cancers and those cancers where the cost-benefit ratio clearly favors drug treatment*". All 17 were developed between 1953 and 1983 and are now generic drugs available at low cost. Several newer, more expensive proprietary drugs probably should be added to this list of efficacious agents, notably Imatinib mesylate and Trastuxumab. Drugs listed by the WHO in a second and third groups, including most of the newer, more expensive drugs, were described as having "*some advantages in certain clinical situations*" and "*not essential for the effective delivery of cancer care*", respectively [46]. Most cancer drugs have anti-proliferative rather than anti-cancer activity, affecting proliferative cells whether normal or cancerous. As a result, their therapeutic window is modest and side effects are the norm. With very few exceptions, most of these drugs were discovered by luck (such as Nitrogen mustard, a by-product of mustard gas), by serendipity (i.e. Mitoxantrone, a derivative of ametantrone, a coal-tar derivative originally intended as an ink), or by trial and error (synthetic analogs of the anthracycline antibiotic Daunorubicin). For decades, agents initially developed to treat infections but discarded because of excessive toxicity, especially to highly proliferative bone marrow and intestine-lining cells, became prime candidates for screening for anti-cancer activity. Early examples of this strategy include Actinomycin D (Dactinomycin) [47], the second antibiotic discovered after Penicillin, and other so-called anti-tumor antibiotics still in use today such as Mitomycin-C, Daunorubicin, Mithramycin, Doxorubicin, Bleomycin, Mitoxantrone, and Idarubicin. At the other extreme of the anti-cancer drug development spectrum, in time and sophistication, are current attempts to design drugs to alter molecular targets pivotal to the proliferative or survival advantage of cancer cells, as exemplified by Gleevec ®.

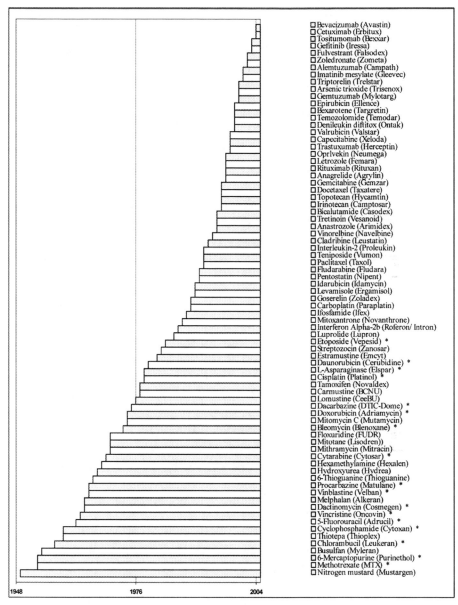

Figure 13. Cancer drugs listed by year of FDA approval or of first clinical trial (* denotes 17 drugs classified as essential by the WHO).

This agent, the first of its kind, is a tyrosine kinase inhibitor that blocks the *bcr/abl* fusion gene-encoded product and in so doing removes the proliferative advantage of chronic myelogenous leukemia cells [48], without cell kill and with little toxicity. Excitement and high expectations followed the 1948 report of the first complete remissions, albeit transient ones, in childhood leukemia treated with folic acid antagonists [39]. Choriocarcinoma became the first curable invasive cancer only five years later [40] and the future of chemotherapy seemed assured. However, failure to replicate these successes in other cancers led researchers to attempt exploiting potential differences between normal and cancer cell biology for therapeutic gain, focusing attention on the cell cycle. This, despite misgivings by a pioneer cancer researcher who warned: "*It is almost, not quite, but almost as hard as finding some agent that will dissolve away the left ear, say, yet leave the right ear unharmed: so slight is the difference between the cancer cell and its normal ancestors*" [50]. Nevertheless, it was discovered that while all cancer drugs seemed to block cell replication, they did so via inhibiting specific phases of the cell cycle (phase-specific drugs), or acting directly or indirectly on DNA, RNA or the cell membrane (not phase-specific drugs). Phase-specific drugs exert their effect either during the S or DNA synthesis phase, the M or mitotic phase, or during the G1 or G2 phases of the cell cycle. Hence, anti-tumor drugs are sub-classified into several distinct categories according to their mechanism of action. They include: 1) Alkylating agents, such as the nitrogen mustards, nitrosoureas, and the platinum subgroups, are not phase-specific drugs but impair cell replication by forming bonds with DNA, RNA and certain proteins. 2) Anti-tumor antibiotics, such as Dactinomycin, Doxorubicin, and Bleomycin are non phase-specific agents with a complex mechanism of action. These agents, best exemplified by the Anthracyclin subgroup, disrupt cell replication by intercalating between base-pairs of DNA disrupting DNA replication and RNA transcription, producing single- and double-stranded DNA splits, damaging DNA through creation of free radicals, and possibly disrupting cell membranes. 3) Antimetabolites, such as Methotrexate, Cytarabine, and 5-fluorouracil, are S-phase specific agents that are structural analogs to normally occurring metabolites involved in DNA synthesis. They exert their cytotoxic activity by competing with metabolites involved in key RNA or DNA regulatory enzymes or by directly substituting metabolites normally incorporated in the RNA or DNA molecules themselves. 4) Mitotic inhibitors, best represented by the vinca alkaloids (Vincristine and Vinblastine) bind tubulin, a cell protein that polymerizes to form the microtubular filaments along which chromosomes migrate during mitosis (cell division). 5) Vinca alkaloids prevent tubulin polymerization resulting in arrest of cell division in metaphase followed by lysis. 6) Finally, a number of older drugs, such as L-asparaginase, and many of the newer ones, such as the monoclonal antibody and the immunotoxins groups, and cancer-active hormones, have mechanisms of action that do not fit into any of these categories. Furthermore, as in any biologic process, the factors and steps involved in cytotoxic cell death are multifaceted and the result of a multitude of contributing intra- and extra-cellular signals, and other factors peculiar to a particular cancer and a given host. For example Fludarabine, an antimetabolite purine analogue that blocks DNA synthesis via inhibiting DNA polymerase alpha, ribonucleotide reductase, and DNA primase, would be expected to exert its greatest activity against cancers with high growth rates. Instead, it is most active against chronic lymphocytic leukemia, a human malignancy characterized by one of the lowest growth rates where the main defect is impaired apoptosis that results in the accumulation of long-lived malignant cells. Additionally, cell cycle kinetics alone fails to describe tumor growth adequately or to explain unexpected tumor response patterns to anti-tumor drugs. Indeed, the cell cycle time for normal cells is 1 to 2 days versus 2 to 3 days in most cancers [49], and the proliferative cell pool in CML is up to 10-fold greater than in acute myeloblastic leukemia (AML) despite its much less aggressive course and much longer survival. The explanation for this apparent incongruity rests on the fact that CML myeloblasts differentiate into mature, functional, and short-lived granulocytes, whereas AML myeloblasts do not differentiate, and, given their high proliferative rate and longer life span, accumulate rapidly [49,50].

Thus, as clinical trial results often failed to confirm anti-tumor drug efficacy predicted by their mechanisms of action and by cell kinetics data, new hypotheses were postulated to explain the observed discrepancies. An early and influential hypothesis was that of Skipper who, based on the L1210 mouse leukemia model, proposed two laws widely regarded as ground-breaking [50]: the first law established that the doubling time of proliferating cancer cells is constant and exponential. The second law postulated that anti-tumor drugs follow "*first-order kinetics*"; that is, the fraction of cells killed by a given drug at a given dose in a given tumor is constant regardless of the size or sate of the cancer. According to this view, a drug that kills 90% of cells of a tumor will do so each time it is administered, whether the tumor is very large or microscopic. However, clinical observations were at variance with Skipper's laws, leading to the Mendelsohn's concept of growth fraction [51] and the hypothesis of Goldie and Coldman on drug resistance [52]. Indeed, most human tumors do not expand exponentially and respond to chemotherapy following patterns far more complex than suggested by a simplistic first order kinetics model.

According to Mendelsohn's concept of growth fraction, tumors are composed of proliferative and non-proliferative cell pools, with the former dictating the growth of the entire tumor and its response to chemotherapy [53]. Mendelsohn's concept of growth fraction provided the kinetic basis for the non-exponential growth pattern of human cancers first proposed by Gompertz in 1825. The Gompertzian tumor growth curve follows a sigmoid pattern with the fastest growth occurring when tumors reach about one third of their final size, and slower growth at both ends of the curve when absolute and relative numbers of proliferative cells, respectively, are few. Thus, in theory very small tumors and micro-metastases should be more sensitive to chemotherapy and easier to eradicate than large tumors. However, clinical observations regarding metastatic recurrences after chemotherapy-induced complete remissions seemed to contradict this postulate, triggering several clinical trials designed to scientifically examine the issue. Of these, perhaps the most convincing was conducted in women with operable breast cancer given adjuvant chemotherapy in attempts to eradicate metastases [54]. After a 10-year follow-up, this study demonstrated that chemotherapy failed to eradicate most metastases, thus supporting the Goldie-Coldman hypothesis on drug resistance. According to this hypothesis, cancer cells mutate with a probability that increases exponentially to tumor size, with mutants often being unresponsive to cancer drugs. Tumors larger than 0.1 cm^3 in size were calculated to be incurable with any single anti-cancer drug.

None of these hypotheses lead to more efficacious cancer management and today the outcome of most cancer patients remains grim, as illustrated by lung cancer, the most lethal malignancy in the US accounting for 28% of all cancer deaths in 2002 [55]. In a retrospective analysis of all randomized phase III clinical trials conducted in North America between 1973 and 1992 on a total of 14,182 patients with advanced lung cancer, prolongation of survival and overall survival remained dismal and unchanged. The survival advantage of patients receiving the experimental drugs rarely exceeded 2 months compared to controls, and median survivals edged up from 5.2 months in the first decade (1973-1983) to 5.8 months in the second (1984-1994). Results were similar whether patients had small cell (SCLC, 5,746) or non-small cell (NSCLC, 8,436) lung cancer. These results, after 22 years of clinical trials involving 24 anti-cancer drugs used singly or in combination, are not only sobering in themselves but, as pointed out by the authors, *"factors that may also have contributed to prolonged survival include improvements in supportive care and general medical management of these patients, in addition to more selective inclusion criteria for trials in more recent years. Improved surgical and imaging staging techniques may have also resulted in the identification and treatment with less extensive 'advanced-stage' disease in more recent years"*. This lack of progress in lung cancer management during this period was confirmed at the national level by SEER data that showed a minimal change in overall median survival from 6.9 months to 7.3 months, and a 3-year survival achieved by a dismal 2% of patients in 1973 that *"rose"* to 4% in 1994 [56]. Since then, no breakthroughs have occurred. Indeed, in a 1998 editorial [58] titled *"The snail's pace of lung cancer therapy"* commemorating the 50th anniversary of Karnofsky's 1948 lung cancer trial that achieved a 49% response rate and a median survival of 5 months in 35 patients treated with Nitrogen mustard [57], the author concluded "*in the past 50 years, the progress in controlling advanced or metastatic lung carcinoma has been slow, but minor improvements have been made*". In 2002, a Cochrane Review [59] reported on a meta-analysis performed on "*all available (52) randomized trials*" that included 9,387 patients with NSCLC, treated with surgery, radiation, or supportive care alone or with adjuvant chemotherapy. Addition of chemotherapy appeared to confer a marginal survival benefit leading the authors to conclude very cautiously, "*These results offer hope of progress and suggest that chemotherapy may have a role in treating this disease*". Finally, the same year a large phase III trial that randomized 1,207 patients with NSCLC to one of four chemotherapy regimens [60] reported 16% to 21% response rates, lasting 3.5 to 4.5 months, and median survivals ranging from 7.4 to 8.3 months. Thus, the number one cancer killer in the US remains essentially unaffected after 52 years of clinical trials assessing the efficacy of most available anti-cancer drugs. Given these sobering facts it is astonishing that a recent review on the cost of NSCLC treatment concluded, "*The available literature suggests that combined modality therapies for locally advanced NSCLC and most chemotherapeutic approaches used in the treatment of metastatic NSCLC fall within the generally accepted definitions of cost-effectiveness*" [61].

Attempts to overcome drug resistance and to enhance anti-tumor drug activity have followed three main paths: Combination of drugs, dose intensity, and high-dose chemotherapy. Multi-drug regimens were developed based on the premise that administration of drugs with non-overlapping mechanisms of action and different dose-limiting toxicities might reduce the emergence of resistant mutants, exhibit greater anti-tumor activity, and be less toxic, [62,63]. Indeed, drug combinations enable administration of each constituent drug at maximum tolerated doses thus increasing the overall therapeutic effects while reducing the likelihood of multi-drug resistant mutants. Numerous drug combinations were tried with varying success until the pioneering regimen known as VAMP (Vincristine, Amethopterin, 6-Mercaptopurine, Prednisone) was developed to treat childhood leukemia [64]. This well-designed regimen incorporated the potential advantages cited above plus intensive, intermittent treatment cycles given over a few days in attempts to achieve high leukemia-cell kill while allowing bone marrow recovery between treatment cycles. The success of this regimen influenced the design of the MOPP protocol (Mustargen ®, Oncovin ®, Prednisone, and Procarbazine) for advanced-stage Hodgkin's disease [65]. In a large study including over 198 patients with mostly advanced stages III and IV Hodgkin's disease, MOPP induced unprecedented 80% complete remission rates and 68% of patients remained disease-free beyond 10 years from the end of the treatment [66]. However, although the concept of combining drugs with different mechanisms of action and non-overlapping toxicities was quickly incorporated into almost all existing chemotherapy regimens, only one potentially curative regimen named PVB (Platinum, Vinblastine, and Bleomycin), this time for testicular cancer [67], proved efficacious and was added to our armamentarium. These isolated successes lead some researchers not to question the appropriateness of this approach or the efficacy of cytotoxic drugs but to recommend escalating drug delivery through *"dose intensity"* and *"high-dose chemotherapy"* as solutions to achieve higher cure rates.

Dose intensity refers to the cumulative dose administered over a prescribed period of time. It was based on the observation that reductions in cumulative dose resulting from dose adjustments or treatment delays lead to falling cure rates in Hodgkin's disease [68], and decreased tumor response rates in breast and colon cancers [69]. The concept of dose intensity was not espoused in the clinical setting perhaps because it implied that chemotherapy regimens as initially designed were somehow therapeutically optimal, but evolved to dose intensification, an age-old notion that drugs are likely to be more effective if administered in high doses. Indeed, arsenic the most widely used anti-cancer agent through the centuries, *"could be given in large, heroic doses for variable periods...*(and that)*...timid doses were only homeopathic and not worthy of consideration"* [70]. Under this scenario the dose was escalated as permitted by the degree of *"epithelial, neurologic or gastrointestinal toxicity"*. A gruesome example of arsenic balm toxicity reported in 1803 described, "*in less than a month, it ate away the breast, the pectoral muscles, the ribs, and the pericardium so that one could see the heart beat for three days, after which she died*" [71]. Two centuries later, the belief that potentially lethal doses of chemotherapy would cure cancer took hold when technological advances enabled administration of bone marrow or peripheral blood stem cells, the purpose of which is to *"rescue"* the most chemotherapy-vulnerable tissue: the bone marrow. Cancer patients treated according to this approach first receive high-dose chemotherapy, sometimes complemented by radiotherapy, which although directed against cancer cells also destroys the highly susceptible bone marrow cells. Then, the patient's damaged bone marrow is "*rescued*" by intravenous infusion of stem cells preserved from the patient's own bone marrow or peripheral blood prior to chemotherapy, or obtained from a matched related or unrelated donor. In the first case, the transplant is called "*autologous*", in the latter, "*allogeneic*". In rare cases where the donor cells derive from the patient's identical twin the transplant is called "*syngeneic*". This "rescue" procedure, made possible by advances in histocompatibility typing methods in the 1960s, evolved from a majority of allogeneic bone marrow transplants in the 1970s and 1980s, to the technically easier and better tolerated autologous peripheral stem cell procedure that predominates today.

High dose chemotherapy with bone marrow or peripheral stem cell rescue enjoyed phenomenal growth in the 1980s and 1990s. For example, in 1999, 21,340 transplants were performed at 580 European transplant centers. Of these, 31% were allogeneic and 69% were autologous. Forty-five percent of allogeneic and 95% of autologous transplants were of blood stem cells. Diseases treated this way included lymphomas (44%), leukemias (34%), solid tumors (18%), and non-malignant, mostly genetic, disorders (4%). While certain subsets of leukemias and lymphomas are benefited by this approach, its impact on solid tumors is still controversial at best despite its high appeal to patients and physicians alike. For example, after preliminary encouraging reports in the early 1990s, breast cancer patients and advocates began demanding this type of treatment, leading some courts to mandate insurance companies to cover the costs of their expensive (up to $100,000) though unproven procedure. Many drives were organized in local communities to raise funds for uninsured breast cancer victims. As a result of public pressure, by the mid-1990s most women with breast cancer were receiving this experimental treatment rather than standard chemotherapy.

Eventually, several randomized studies were begun in the late 1990s. Preliminary results from four of five breast cancer studies in America, Europe, and South Africa have shown that high-dose chemotherapy plus bone marrow rescue confers no survival advantage over conventional chemotherapy. In the largest of these studies, conducted by the Cancer and Leukemia Group B, 784 women with metastatic breast cancer were first treated with four cycles of conventional chemotherapy and then randomized to either high dose chemotherapy plus blood stem cell rescue, or to intermediate dose chemotherapy. All women whose tumor status was hormone receptor positive or unknown received radiation therapy to the chest and Tamoxifen. Disease-free and overall survivals at three years were equivalent for both groups. There was a slight reduction in relapses (20% vs. 28%) but a higher death rate (7.4% vs. 0%) in women receiving high dose chemotherapy with blood stem cell rescue [72]. In another two trials involving 533 and 525 women with breast cancer, one conducted by the Eastern Cooperative Oncology Group, the other in Scandinavia, no survival advantage was demonstrated for women treated with high-dose chemotherapy plus autologous stem-cell transplantation when compared to women receiving conventional-dose chemotherapy [73]. Likewise, the French study showed no difference in the two groups of women in terms of progression-free or overall survival. The only positive study was conducted at the University of Witwatersrand in South Africa. However, inconsistencies in the records lead to a formal audit at the request of the

South African Medical Research Council and the University of Witwatersrand which found unequivocal evidence of scientific misconduct and falsified data that lead to a formal retraction of the published data [74]. A meta-analysis [75] of nine randomized trials involving 3,525 breast cancer patients, published in 2004, concluded that high-dose chemotherapy plus bone marrow or stem cell transplant offers no substantial survival advantage at 3 or 5 years over conventional chemotherapy. This, despite more frequent and more severe side-effects and worse quality of life immediately after treatment. Thus, based on this cumulative experience, it has been suggested that high-dose chemotherapy plus marrow or stem cell transplant should not be the standard of care.

The use of high-dose chemotherapy in other malignancies has also disappointed. In multiple myeloma it does not prolong survival when compared to treatment with drugs available in the mid-1960s; autologous stem-cell transplantation is of marginal survival benefit, and despite a 40% mortality rate allogeneic transplantation is not curative [76]. Likewise, in a retrospective analysis of 1,036 patients who had undergone bone marrow transplantation for leukemia, lymphoma, and genetic disorders, the long-term incidence of second malignancies was 3.8-fold higher than in age-matched controls [77]. Thus, high dose chemotherapy with bone marrow or blood stem cell rescue has not only failed to deliver on the high expectations of its proponents but might be associated with unforeseen long-term complications.

Although multi-drug regimens, dose intensity, and high-dose chemotherapy proved to be largely unsuccessful strategies to overcome drug resistance and to enhance anti-tumor activity, their foundations were cogent when first enunciated. However, some proposals bordered on the fanciful and whimsical as exemplified by "*chronotherapy*". This hypothesis theorized that the efficacy and toxicity of cancer drugs vary with human circadian rhythms. This idea led adhering oncologists to administer chemotherapy at odd hours of the day and night expecting enhanced efficacy and reduced toxicity. It also encouraged the emergence of electronic pumps and devices capable of delivering drugs at preset times, rates, and following certain patterns designed to harmonize with the patient's "*biorhythms*". In a relatively recent chemotherapy textbook [78], the longest of its 61 chapters addressed "*Circadian timing and toxicity*" and concluded passionately "*This medical movement toward temporal considerations will abolish the separate science of chronobiology and ultimately make all biologists and physicians chronobiologists*".

This brief discussion of the evolution of cancer chemotherapy leads to the conclusion that given their non-specificity and narrow therapeutic window, the anticancer activity of cytotoxic drugs reached a low efficacy plateau that could not be breached by dose escalation, drug combination, timing or schedule of administration, or by other manipulations. As a result and despite the most assiduous and lengthy efforts by the largest number of researchers ever assembled to conquer a disease, most advanced cancers respond only marginally to cytotoxic chemotherapy drugs, as discussed below.

Chapter 7

TREATMENT OUTCOMES: DISMAL BY ANY STANDARD

What has the cell-kill paradigm and its dominance of cancer research, diagnosis, treatment, and outcome assessment achieved in the context of the *War on cancer* since the enactment of the National Cancer Act of 1971? The answer will vary depending on how achievement is measured and who does the assessment. For example, in a 1996 review article titled *The war on cancer* [79] marking the 25th birthday of the National Cancer Act of 1971, the author used a quote from Charles Dickens to dramatize its failure: "*Dead, your Majesty. Dead, my lords and gentlemen. Dead, right reverends and wrong reverends of every order. Dead, men and women, born with Heavenly compassion in your hearts. And dying thus around us every day*". Less than a year later, an editorial written by a former Director of the NCI rejoiced "*Happy birthday 'War', you deserve a pat on the back*" [80]. Both authors converged on crediting major scientific advances made during this period, especially the breathtaking advances in molecular biology and molecular genetics, including the genome project, that have revolutionized our knowledge about cancer. Yet, while both see a brighter future after these advances are applied to the practice of medicine, the former author concluded "*We must develop new approaches to control this plague of deaths, adopting an ethic of prevention ....to prevent disease before it becomes invasive and metastatic*" [79].

In order to determine which of these opposing views is supported by the facts, progress against cancer must be measured objectively and factually. Direct measurements of progress include changes in incidence and mortality rates and in duration and quality of life after diagnosis [81]. However, interpretation of changing trends in these outcomes must take into account a host of impacting factors that are tangential to the management of cancer.

Some of the most obvious confounding factors include, early-stage and slow-growing tumors, "*stage migration*", and overall improvements in health care. For example, increasing numbers of early-stage and slow-growing tumors fostered by screening have contributed to rising incidence rates and improved survival, as in the case of breast and prostate cancer. Likewise, refinements in cancer staging techniques have contributed to *stage migration* over time. That is, patients with occult metastases undetected in the era preceding computer-assisted tomography and magnetic resonance imaging (MRI) were classified as having local or regional disease whereas they are now included in the advanced stage category. As a result of their removal from the group of localized disease and their inclusion in the group of advanced disease, the average survival for both groups has risen. This is because fewer of these patients with poor prognosis are included in the former group and the later now includes patients with "*early*" advanced disease (based on CT or MRI staging), whereas in the past it was populated by patients with clinically far-advanced or symptomatic disease. Improvements in general medical support measures such as potent antibiotics to treat chemotherapy-associated infections, easier access to blood product transfusions, and other life-sustaining measures all contribute to surviving previously fatal treatment complications. Because trends in cancer incidence have already been examined in chapters 1 and 2, the discussion that follows will analyze cure rates, the outcome least influenced by factors peripheral to cancer treatment per se, cancer mortality, cancer survival, and quality of life. The analysis will concentrate on national trends over time, for they are the barometers that mirror progress in cancer treatment and cancer control, and ultimately gauge the success or failure of the *War on Cancer*. Because the subject of this book is Medical Oncology, the focus will be on invasive and metastatic cancers treated with chemotherapy.

First, we must recognize that "*cure*" is not an absolute term because minimal residual or slowly recurrent disease that causes no symptoms can persist and remain undetected for years. This is because cancer-specific detection tools exist for but a few cancers and non-specific tests available to assess the status of most cancers are insufficiently sensitive to detect minimal residual disease in the absence of symptoms or signs of recurrence. For example, while leukemias can be assessed at the cellular and molecular levels on easily accessible blood and bone marrow specimens, such highly discriminant detection tools are not available for most cancers. Furthermore, residual and early recurrent asymptomatic cancers other than leukemias are often deeply seated and rely on cruder techniques, such CT-scans and MRI for their detection as a prelude to obtaining a tissue specimen for pathologic confirmation. Given these limitations the consensus is that, for most patients and in most circumstances, a continuous disease-free survival lasting 5 years or longer after completion of treatment is a strong indication that a recurrence will not occur. Using this definition of cure, eleven types of disseminated or metastatic cancers, out of more than 200 known to exist, are considered potentially curable (Table VII); eight treated by chemotherapy alone, and three when treatment combines regional surgery or irradiation supplemented by chemotherapy (called *"adjuvant"* under these circumstances). The actual cure rates, that range from approximately 25% for acute myelocytic leukemia to nearly 90% for gestational choriocarcinoma, are impacted by host factors such as age and presence of co-morbidity, and characteristics of the cancer especially stage and biologic behavior. As shown on Table VII, the overall combined frequency of potentially curable cancers in the US were fewer than 55,000 cases in 2003 (approximately 4% of all cancers), and fewer than 50% of them (or approximately 1.8% of all cancers) will achieve a 5-year survival, disease-free, a figure little changed over two decades.

Table VII. Potentially curable advanced cancers, US 2003.

1. Treated with chemotherapy alone			
Cancer type	*New cases**	*Cure rate (%)#*	*Cured cases***
Trophoblastic cancers	422	90	380
Germ cell cancers	7,600	65	4,940
Leukemias:			
Childhood Lymphoblastic	3,600	75	2,700
Adult:			
Acute Myeloblastic	10,500	25	2,625
Prolymphocytic	100	?	?
Hairy-cell	630	80	504
Hodgkin's disease	7,600	65	4,940
Diffuse large-cell lymphoma	22,480	30	6,744
2. Treated with chemotherapy used as adjuvant			
Cancer type			
Wilms tumor	460	65	299
Osteogenic sarcoma	750	65	488
Rhabdomyosaroma	250	70	175
Totals cases	54,392		23,794
Percent of total US cases ##	4.08		1.78

* New case estimates according to the American Cancer society projections, US 2003.
# Percent cure rates reflect 5-year disease-free survival as reported in the medical literature.
**, Cured cases are new cases times percentage cured rates.
Potentially curable and cured cases expressed as percent of new cases, US 2003

The 2002 *"Annual Report to the Nation on the status of cancer, 1973-1999"* [82] announced, *"Across all ages, overall cancer death rates decreased in men and women from 1993 through 1999"*. This report, prepared in collaboration by NCI, the American Cancer Society, the North American Association of Central Cancer Registries, the National Institute on Aging (NIA), and the Centers for Disease Control and Prevention, was widely quoted by the scientific and popular press. News of decreasing overall cancer mortality rates after 1992 was welcome news and implied that the *War on Cancer* was on the right track. However, the report focused on a favorable period of declining mortality rates that was short-lived, can be credited to prevention and screening measures rather than treatment, and did not extend beyond 2000. In contrast, an analysis of mortality rates between 1973 and 1997 is far more sobering. This time period was chosen because is has the dual advantages of been less prone to short-term fluctuations and to coincide with the enormous resources unleashed by the National Cancer Act of 1971 that launched the *War on Cancer*. Between 1973 and 1997, cancer incidence and mortality rates increased for nine of the most frequent cancers. They were: esophagus, liver, lung and bronchus, melanoma of skin, prostate, kidney and renal pelvis, brain and other nervous system, non-Hodgkin's lymphoma, and multiple myeloma. Together these cancers accounted for 274,209 deaths, or 51% of the total cancer deaths (539,566) in 1997. In contrast, cancers with both decreased incidence and decreased mortality rates [26] (oral cavity and pharynx, stomach, colon and rectum, pancreas, larynx, uterine cervix, uterine corpus, Hodgkin's disease, and leukemias) accounted for 141,747 deaths, or 26% of all cancer deaths in 1997. Cancers with increasing incidence but decreasing mortality rates during that period (breast, ovary, testis, urinary bladder, and thyroid), accounted for 68,571 or 13% of all cancer deaths in 1997. There were no cancers associated with decreasing incidence but increasing mortality rates. Thus, by 1997 there were fewer cancers with decreasing mortality rates (39% of total cancer deaths) than with rising mortality rates (51%). Furthermore, 86% of the decline in average mortality rates was due to reduced deaths rates in only 4 cancers: lung, prostate, colon, and breast [83], and most of the decline is due to smoking cessation, early stage diagnosis, and to improvements in overall health care. Finally, falling overall incidence and death rates after there peaks in the early 1990s were transient as revealed by "*The Annual Report to the Nation on the Status of Cancer 1975-2000*"[84]. The report disclosed no further declines in incidence rates after 1995 or in mortality rates after 1998.

Survival prolongation, even when cancer persists, is also considered a measure of treatment success that can justify the toxicity and costs associated with chemotherapy. True prolongation of survival has been achieved over the last decade or so in subsets of patients afflicted by some cancers including breast, prostate, and colon. On the other hand, favorable survival trends in many cancers observed over several decades relate to factors other than cancer treatment, as discussed earlier.

Finally, given the meager impact of chemotherapy on cancer cure, mortality, and survival rates and a more proactive attitude on the part of patients, the attention of researchers and clinicians was recently turned to quality of life (QOL) as a desirable alternate goal of cancer management [85]. QOL is defined by the World Health Organization as *"not only the lack of infirmity but also a state of physical, mental, and social well being"*. While QOL is an intuitively easy notion to grasp and define in broad terms, it is a multidimensional, dynamic, and subjective concept impacted by psychological, spiritual, personal, familial, and social issues that affect each patient differently [86]. Additionally, the attitudes of healthy individuals, nurses, and physicians towards chemotherapy differ substantially from those of cancer patients' who, facing issues of life and death, are likely to perceive treatment benefits through a prism of hope and high expectations and to embrace any treatment that offers some respite, however slight [87]. Hence, no consensus has been reached on how to objectively assess and quantify QOL or how to design treatment protocols with QOL outcome goals. As a result, clinical trials focused on QOL remain limited in scope or uneven in quality, and more importantly, unable to provide concrete answers. Ideally, the pursuit of a cure, survival prolongation, or improved QOL should not be viewed as mutually exclusive but as concurrent goals in the context of treatment outcome. That is, a temporary assault of the patient's QOL by cytotoxic chemotherapy expected to cure or meaningfully prolong survival is amply justified. In contrast, this is not the case for most cancers where the negative impact of chemotherapy on QOL is not counterbalanced by a favorable patient outcome. Notwithstanding this self-evident principle, in practice QOL is often invoked by tumor-focused physicians to justify to themselves and their despondent patients, the use of inefficacious chemotherapy oblivious of the fact that such decisions usually lead to more suffering without mitigating benefits. More on this later.

In conclusion, an objective analysis of cancer chemotherapy outcomes over the last three decades reveals that, despite vast human and financial expenditures, the cell-killing paradigm has failed to achieve its objective [88], the former rallying phrase *War on Cancer* has been abandoned by the NCI, and the conquest of cancer remains a distant and elusive goal. Moreover, as long as the use of inefficacious but toxic drugs is justified by the exigencies of the cell-kill paradigm, a model based on flawed premises with an unattainable goal, cytotoxic chemotherapy in its present form will neither eradicate cancer nor alleviate suffering. Moreover, if perpetuated this approach would continue to divert vast financial and human resources, and sequester the efforts of well-meaning though misguided clinical researchers and the attention of policy-makers, thus postponing the adoption of cogent cancer control policies. In the meantime, aware of the ineffectiveness and toxicity of today's chemotherapy drugs, desperate cancer patients seek providers of "*alternative medicine*", who at best dispense harmless but inefficacious compounds, or at worst are unscrupulous charlatans who combine a profit motive to a profound disregard for patients' welfare.

PART IV

WHY DOES THIS SYSTEM PERSIST?

In the previous chapter I presented evidence that the three crucial measures of progress in the War on Cancer, cure rates, prolongation of survival, and quality of life, remain stagnant despite enactment of the National Cancer Act of 1971. I have also shown that, in large measure, this stagnation results from an unbalanced focus on treatment of inoperable cancer to the detriment of prevention and early detection, and adherence to the infectious disease model that has driven drug development towards the cancer cell-kill paradigm. Based on these considerations I advanced the notion that, given their non-specificity and narrow therapeutic window, such drugs have not and will not achieve the desired results. While others have previously questioned the status or direction of the *War on Cancer*, they have done so mostly within the confines of the scientific community [1-3] or have publicly denounced or implied a conspiracy among players in the cancer field [4], a position that merits little credibility. So, why does the system persist year after year, decade after decade? Why have so few voices decried this state of affairs? The answers to these questions are complex but can be found in an analysis of the entrenched views, perceptions, and motivations of the major players that directly or indirectly impact clinical cancer research and patient management, as described in the next 4 chapters.

Chapter 8

THE ROLE OF THE NATIONAL CANCER INSTITUTE

1.   HISTORICAL BACKGROUND

From the legislative standpoint, today's National Cancer Institute (NCI) is an outgrowth of several attempts by the US Congress that culminated in the National Cancer Institute Act of 1937. Earlier Congressional attempts to address cancer were disorganized, uncoordinated, ill conceived, and naive mainly because of the very limited knowledge and the misconceptions of the time regarding cancer. For example, on February 4, 1927 Senator Mathew M. Neely of West Virginia introduced the first cancer bill (S 5589) "*to authorize a reward* (5 million dollars) *for the discovery of a successful cure for cancer, and to create a commission to inquire into and ascertain the success of such a cure*". This approach, reminiscent of the legendary wild west reward for the head of a fugitive, triggered a deluge of bizarre claims by the usual assortment of quacks, snake-oil healers, and other profit-motivated, unsavory characters. However, ten years and several similar misguided bills later, Congressman Maury Maverick introduced, on April 29, 1937, bill HR 6767, "*to promote research in the cause, prevention, and methods of diagnosis and treatment of cancer, to establish a National Cancer Center in the Public Health Service, and for other purposes*". In drafting the bill, which ultimately placed the proposed National Cancer Center within the Public Health Service, Congressman Maverick received legal advice from the Public Health Service and expert medical guidance from Dr. Dudley Jackson, of San Antonio, Texas. After reconciling competing views regarding its mission and structure, the National Cancer Act, PL 244 with an annual budget of $700,000, was passed by a joint committee of Congress on

July 23, 1937, and signed into law by President Franklin D. Roosevelt on August 5 of the same year. The first Director of the new institute, who was to report directly to the US Surgeon General, was Carl Voegtlin, head of Pharmacology at the Public Health Service. Voegtlin merged his group with researchers at the Office of Cancer Investigations of Harvard University to establish the first core of researchers at the new NCI, and issued the first thirteen research fellowship grants. Construction of the first independent home for the NCI began in June 1939 and was dedicated with great fanfare by President Roosevelt on October 31, 1940, to house the Institute's first one hundred staff members. That same year, Voegtlin launched the Journal of the National Cancer Institute, serving as its first editor. However, despite numerous legislative, organizational, and research initiatives, the overall impact of the NCI on cancer survival over the ensuing 30 years was minimal.

On April 27, 1970, at the urging of the chairman of the Senate Labor and Public Welfare Committee, Senator Ralph W. Yarborough ("*the People's Senator*" [5]), the Senate approved the creation of the National Panel of Consultants on the Conquest of Cancer. On November 25, 1970, seven months after receiving its mandate, the Panel submitted to the Senate its report entitled "*National Program for the Conquest of Cancer*". The power behind the entire project was cancer activist Mary Lasker, a New Yorker and wife of advertising magnate Albert Lasker. The Laskers were philanthropic supporters of the American Cancer Society who had established the Lasker Foundation in 1942 to promote health care research through yearly Awards that honor prominent basic science and clinical researchers. After her husband's death from colon cancer in 1952, Mary became convinced that only the resources of the Federal government could confront the cancer challenge. Using her extensive network of political, business, medical, and social contacts, and the considerable financial resources of her husband's estate, ironically bolstered by an advertising campaign to convince women to smoke ("*Reach for a Lucky instead of a sweet*"), Mary launched an assault on cancer. If American ingenuity was capable of putting a man on the moon in a decade, the conquest of cancer seemed an attainable goal by the nation's Bicentennial. However, her access to the Kennedy's White House facilitated by partially funding Jacqueline Kennedy's redecoration project and the expansive spending of Lyndon Johnson's government came to an end when Richard M. Nixon became President. Given Nixon's preoccupation with inflation and pressures on the US Congress to limit spending, she adopted a two-prong strategy: she surrounded herself with high-profile researchers such as Sidney Farber, Scientific Director of the Children's Cancer Research Foundation in Boston and former President of the American Cancer Society, and business leaders such as Benno Schmidt, an investment banker who would later co-Chair with Farber the Senate's National Panel of Consultants. She also befriended influential politicians, especially Senator Yarborough, chairman of the powerful Senate Labor and Public Welfare Committee. Farber, who in the 1940s reported the first remissions in acute childhood leukemia [6], believed, as did Solomon Garb author of the book Cure for Cancer [7], that the cure of cancer could be achieved with little further research, if concerted efforts and sufficient funds were allocated to its eradication. Likewise, Randolph L. Clark, a cancer researcher and editor of the YearBook of Cancer declared, *"With a billion dollars a year for ten years we could lick cancer"*. Farber argued before the Senate Labor and Public Welfare Committee, *"The 325,000 patients with cancer who are going to die this year cannot wait; nor is it necessary, in order to make great progress in the cure of cancer, for us to have the full solution of all the problems of basic research....the history of Medicine is replete with examples of cures obtained years, decades, and even centuries before the mechanism of action was understood for these cures"* [8].

Farber's views were not shared by many including some of his own colleagues at Harvard such as Francis Moore, surgeon-in-chief at the Peter Bent Brigham Hospital, in Boston. Moore correctly argued that most breakthroughs in medical science have originated from creative, independent researchers, not from organized, centrally-directed research as was being proposed. Likewise, many National Institutes of Health (NIH) researchers were privately dismayed at Farber's views, and at the goals being set they knew to be unattainable within the timeframe contemplated. Additionally, the medical establishment was vehemently opposed to the plan arguing that a cancer program outside the NIH would be isolated from other biomedical research potentially useful in the fight against cancer. In order to prevail despite mounting objections from skeptics and critics, Lasker organized a grass-roots cancer advocacy group called the Citizens' Committee for the Conquest of Cancer. In December 1969 her committee initiated a public-relation campaign aimed at influencing the US Senate, where the National Cancer Act, a bill she also spear-headed, was being debated. A full-page advertisement published on December 9, 1969 by the New York Times read *"Mr. Nixon: You can cure cancer. If prayers are heard in Heaven, this prayer is heard the most, 'Dear God, please, not cancer'. Still more than 318,000 Americans died of cancer last year. This year, Mr. President, you have it in your power to begin to end this curse."* Other ads read *"This year, Mr. President, we are so close to the cure of cancer. We lack only the will and the kind of money....that went into putting a man on the moon. Why don't we try to conquer cancer by America's 200th birthday?"*. Moreover, she enlisted the help of her good friend syndicated columnist Ann Landers who urged her readers to write lawmakers in support of the bill. An estimated

300,000 letters landed at Congress' doorsteps as it debated the merits of the National Cancer Act. Members of the Senate Labor and Public Welfare Committee opposing the bill received individual letters threatening that their reelection would be opposed if they did not reconsider their opposition to the cancer act.

President Nixon embraced the cancer cause and in his January 22, 1971 State of the Union address declared: *"The time has come in America when the same kind of concentrated effort that split the atom and took man to the moon should be turned toward conquering this dread disease. Let us make a total national commitment to achieve this goal. America has long been the wealthiest nation in the world. Now it is time we became the healthiest nation in the world"* [9]. He converted, in October 1971, the Army's Fort Detrick, in Maryland from a biological warfare facility to a national cancer research center, now called the Frederick Cancer Research and Development Center. In the meantime, Senator Edward Kennedy had become Committee Chairman and co-sponsor of the final bill when Senator Yarborough lost his bid for reelection in 1970. Fearing that Kennedy might oppose him in the presidential race of 1972, President Nixon, who had lost the presidential race to John F. Kennedy in 1960, opposed the Kennedy name on that important legislation. Eventually, Senator Kennedy withdrew his name as sponsor of the bill and President Nixon signed into law the National Cancer Act on December 23, 1971, stating: *"I hope in the years ahead we will look back on this action today as the most significant taken during my Administration"* [9]. The law established the NCI within the NIH but with a budget to be submitted directly to the President for approval, thus bypassing the NIH and the Department of Health, Education, and Welfare. Its director became a presidential appointee. The Act also created a President's Cancer Panel, composed of two scientists and one management specialist who would submit to the President yearly progress reports on the status of research at NCI. The act also replaced the National Advisory Cancer Council with an eighteen-member National Cancer Advisory Board of scientists and laypersons empowered to guide and advise the NCI on all initiatives [10]. Since then, numerous amendments and other legislative actions have complemented and expanded the National Cancer Program according to constituent needs and political pressures. These include the Community Mental Health Center Extension, and the Biomedical Research and Research Training Amendments of 1978, and the NIH Revitalization Amendments of 1993. As a result, the NCI budget has grown from $492.2 million in 1973 to $4,770.5 billion in 2004 [12], or a nearly 8% average annual increase after inflation.

2. CURRENT ORGANIZATION, ROLE, AND INFLUENCE

According to its own vision the NCI *"conducts, coordinates, and funds cancer research and provides vision and leadership for the cancer research community by: Planning and prioritizing all aspects of the research we support; conducting ongoing assessments to ensure a comprehensive and balanced research portfolio; seeking advice regularly from our stakeholders; supporting core extramural and intramural programs; and maintaining a strong infrastructure to support cancer research"* [10]. This mandate is exercised through its two key programs: the Extramural Research Program, which links the NCI to a myriad of off-site investigators at academic institutions, research centers, and other sites throughout the country and the Intramural Research Program, which encompasses the work of over 4,000 researchers, clinicians and staff employed by NCI. The NCI's Extramural Research Program includes five areas: the Division of Cancer Biology that *"ensures continuity and stability in basic cancer research while encouraging and facilitating the emergence of new ideas, concepts, technologies and possibilities"*; the Division of Cancer Control and Population Sciences, that *"aims to reduce risk, incidence, and deaths from cancer as well as enhance the quality of life for cancer survivors"*; the Division of Cancer Treatment and Diagnosis (DCTD) that *"through a national program of funding cancer research, improves the lives of the American public by discovering better ways to detect, assess, cure and control cancer"*; and the Division of Extramural Activities with a mandate to *"coordinate the scientific review of extramural research before funding, and to provide systematic surveillance of that research after awards are made"*. The NCI's Intramural Research Program includes the Center for Cancer Research (CCR) and the Division of Cancer Epidemiology and Genetics (DCEG). The CCR emerged from the 2001 merger of the Divisions of Basic and Clinical Research. As the largest NCI program the CCR takes advantage of its 329 Principal Investigators in 54 Laboratories, Branches, and Programs to *"foster interdisciplinary programs and facilitate translational research"*; The DCEG *"plans, directs, manages, and evaluates"* the NCI's intramural program of epidemiology, demographic, biostatistical, and population-based genetic research.

In conclusion, given its enormous and ever increasing budget and reach, the NCI has the financial resources to, and does in fact, fund most of the nation's non-private cancer research at any given time. This financial muscle, backed by an excellent and far-reaching organizational infrastructure, gives the NCI the power to *"plan, prioritize, direct, coordinate, evaluate, administer, and serve as the focal point"* for most of the nation's basic and applied cancer research. It is ironic that the country that stands the tallest among nations for free flow of ideas leads its *War on Cancer* through a central bureaucracy whose mandate is to control the type and direction of nearly all cancer research. Thus, given its extraordinary influence on the direction of basic and applied cancer research, the NCI must be credited for the nation's advances in molecular biology and genetics of cancer but should also be held accountable for three decades of stagnation in cancer treatment.

3.   CANCER CENTERS PROGRAM

In 1961, the NIH established three new grant programs aimed at fostering cancer research in the United States. They included the Cancer research Facilities Grants, the Program Project Grants, and the Cancer Clinical Research Center Grants, that were intended to support broad-based institutional and individual basic and applied cancer research. But it was the National Cancer Act of 1971 that broadened the Centers mandate and scope to include research, patient care, training and education, and cancer control. The intended multidisciplinary approach to Cancer Centers was patterned after well-established models such as Roswell Park Cancer Institute in Buffalo, NY, M.D. Anderson Cancer Center in Houston, Texas, and Memorial Sloan-Kettering Cancer Center, in New York City. However, evolution of the model has led to the current stratification of Cancer Centers into three categories: Comprehensive Cancer Centers, a category that identifies major academic or research institutions for the depth and breath of their cancer program in basic and applied research, and in the areas of prevention, control, and population-based research; Clinical Cancer Centers that have active applied cancer research and can have research programs in one other area as well; and Cancer Centers, that are organizations with narrowly focused cancer research not involving human subjects. In 2003, NCI supported a total of 61 Centers in 32 States, including 39 Comprehensive Cancer Centers, 14 Clinical Cancer Centers, and 8 Cancer Centers at a cost of $267.4 million [11], or 5.8% of its annual budget. With 9 Centers, California had the most, followed by New York State with 7. It is noteworthy that, in contrast, NCI's Intramural Research Program cost $648.2 million in 2003 [11], or 14.1% of its total budget.

4.   COOPERATIVE TRIALS STRUCTURE

At the urging of Sydney Farber, Mary Lasker, and other cancer advocates, Congress launched the Chemotherapy National Service Center in

1955 with an annual budget of $5 million. This initiative evolved into today's Cooperative Trials Structure (CTS), which includes the Cooperative Clinical Research Program (CCRP) and the Community Clinical Oncology Program (CCOP). Through these programs the CTS funds *"organizations which continually generate and conduct new clinical trials consistent with national priorities for cancer treatment research"*. The term organizations refers to groups of universities and cancer center researchers (CCRP), and community physicians (CCOP) in the United States, Canada, and Europe with a common purpose: to conduct trials in multi-institutional settings aimed at finding *"better ways to prevent, diagnose, or treat cancer"*. The scope of clinical trials is broad: disease-oriented such as the National Wilms' Tumor Study Group or the National Surgical Adjuvant Breast and Bowel Project; focused on gender or age groups such as the Gynecologic Oncology Group and the Pediatric Oncology Group, respectively; or is centered on treatment modality such as the Radiation Therapy Oncology Group and the American College of Surgeons Oncology Group. Finally, the largest groups engage mostly in drug studies encompassing a broad range of cancers and include: the Cancer and Leukemia Group B (CALGB), the Eastern Cooperative Oncology Group (ECOG), the European Organization for Research and Treatment of Cancer (EORCT), and the Southwest Oncology Group (SWOG). Each year, approximately 20,000 new patients, or approximately 2% of the total number of newly diagnosed cancer patients in participating countries, are enrolled (accrued) in one of many available trials. In early 2003, 767 chemotherapy trials in all phases of drug development (233 phase I, 427 phase II and 107 phase III), and for all types of cancer, were sponsored by the NCI to enroll cancer patients in many countries, at a cost of $252.5 million, or 5.5% of NCI's total 2003 operating budget [11].

Traditionally, clinical cancer trials in the US have been sponsored and funded by NCI's DCTD, with its Cancer Therapy Evaluation Program (CTEP) division designing and implementing the development plans for new cancer drugs. However, propelled by the promise of the Human Genome Project, the pharmaceutical industry has more recently taken an increasingly prominent role in sponsoring and funding such trials accounting for most anticancer drugs being developed today. Additionally, collaboration between DCTD and private industry is frequent and, *"since DCTD does not market drugs...the involvement of a private firm is sought as early in development as possible... (to) permit substantial cost-sharing between public and private sectors that can hasten by several years the availability of effective drugs for all cancer patients"*. Through a massive effort involving Cooperative Groups, Cancer Centers, and a multitude of contractors, NCI supports over 7,000 investigators at approximately 1,000 participant institutions. Reliance on clinical trials to assess the therapeutic value and toxicity of new drugs for any disease or condition is so widespread that applications for any drug approval by the US Food and Drug Administration requires submission of scientific data gathered via clinical trials. As a result, incorporation of clinical trials in experimental therapeutics as a prelude to official sanction and widespread drug use can be viewed as one of the major advances in modern medicine, especially as it pertains to the promotion and safeguard of public health.

This approach of using the scientific method to assess the potential benefit of new drugs via human trials, we now take for granted, was first proposed by French physician Pierre Charles Alexandre Louis in 1834. In a treatise entitled Essays in Clinical Instruction [13], Louis advocated the numerical method to assess the benefit of therapies when he wrote "*It is necessary to account for different circumstances of age, sex, temperament, physical condition, natural history of the disease, and errors in giving therapy*". Anticipating resistance to his scientific approach to medicine, he wrote "*The only reproach which can be made to the numerical method is that it offers real difficulties in its execution...it requires much more labor and time than the most distinguished members of our profession can dedicate to it*". His demonstration that resorting to bleeding for treating pneumonia was an illusion sanctioned by theory, tradition, and personal perception rather than by scientific proof [14], was hailed as "*one of the most important medical works of the present century, marking the start of a new era in science*" by the editor of the American Journal of Medical Sciences, where his article was published. It was, he added with remarkable foresight, "*the first formal exposition of the results of the only true method of investigation in regard to the therapeutic value of remedial agents*". At first, Louis' method encountered fierce resistance for physicians were unwilling to have their therapeutic decisions held in limbo until sanctioned by the numerical method, nor were they prepared to discard treatments sanctioned by tradition and by their own perception and personal preference. Skeptical academics held that "*Averages could not help and might even confuse practicing physicians as they struggle to apply general rules to a specific case*". One and a half centuries later many physicians remain suspicious of medical statistics, validating the adage "*plus ça change, plus ça reste la même chose*" (the more it changes the more it stays the same). However, when practitioners recognized that Louis' numerical method enhanced rather than hindered their clinical skills and brought objectivity to their therapeutic choices, his method gained increasing acceptance, and eventually became the norm to assess and validate the usefulness of new and old therapies. Louis attracted many notable foreign disciples, including William Osler who spearheaded adoption of his mentor's method in America. Today, Louis is considered the direct or indirect mentor of most American and English scientists in public health, epidemiology, medicine, and biostatistics.

5.   CLINICAL TRIALS: TYPES, PHASES, DESIGN, AND INTERPRETATION

In order to understand how is cancer research translated into patient care, and how it impacts the *War on Cancer* it is necessary to have an understanding of the nature of clinical cancer trials, especially how they are designed, conducted, and interpreted. Clinical trials are the final stages in the long process of evaluating the positive and negative biological effects of an agent potentially useful in the prevention, diagnosis, or treatment of cancer. Thus, there are three types of clinical trials according to their purpose: Preventive, Diagnostic, and Therapeutic. While they differ somewhat in design, this section will focus on the treatment trial model, and more specifically chemotherapy trials.

Potential anti-cancer drugs are evaluated in successive steps called phases. This process enables researchers to assess in an orderly and sequential fashion the safety (phase I) and activity of a drug administered alone (phase II) or in combination with other drugs (phase III). In phase I trials, a new drug is administered for the first time to humans with the purpose of determining its toxicity at various doses and schedules, when administered orally or parenterally (intravenously or intramuscularly). Thus, the only purpose of phase I trials, which take an average of 1.5 years to complete and enroll between 20 to 100 individuals, is to determine whether a drug has an "*acceptable*" level of toxicity. The term acceptable is crucial but relative, for a relatively high level of toxicity that is acceptable to treat a resistant cancer will be unacceptable to treat a type of responsive cancer for which other beneficial therapies exist. As a result, and from a strategic standpoint, most patients entered into phase I trials have cancers that have proven refractory to standard therapies. If a drug successfully completes phase I trials it will proceed to phase II, a process that enrolls between 100 and 500 patients and averages 2 years to complete. The goals of phase II trials are primarily to establish anti-cancer activity using doses, schedules, and routes of administration associated with acceptable toxicity, and secondarily to further assess toxicity. Patients entered into phase II trials are usually of two categories: patients with refractory cancers and to a lesser extent newly diagnosed patients with advanced cancers known to be habitually unresponsive to established therapies. Once a phase II is successfully completed, the new drug is eligible to proceed to the next phase. In phase III trials, which are always comparative trials involving 1,000 to 5,000 patients and take on the average 3.5 years to complete, the new drug, administered alone or in combination with other standard drugs, is compared side by side to the anti-cancer activity and toxicity of the standard therapy for the type of cancer under study. Thus, one set of patients is assigned the new drug (the experimental group) while a group of comparable patients (the control group) receives the standard drug regimen.

The design of clinical trials is extremely important. It must ensure that differences observed between groups with respect to anti-cancer activity and toxicity are drug-related and not due to dissimilarities in demographic or biological variables, as discovered by Louis 165 years ago. This is because, contrary to the physical sciences where experiments can be reproduced with little variation, clinical research is adversely impacted by the vast heterogeneity of human biology and by the wide range of responses humans often exhibit to the same drug. Given the law of probabilities, two very large groups composed of thousands of individuals each should be nearly homogeneous with respect to distribution by age, sex, and other major variables, rendering them comparable. However, this is not the case in individual clinical trials where the total number of patients enrolled seldom exceeds a few hundred individuals. Moreover, given their high cost and labor-intense execution, and the need for swift enrollment and long follow up of substantial numbers of patients, most phase III clinical trials are conducted in a multi-institutional setting, thus increasing patient heterogeneity and variation in protocol execution. Under these circumstances, particular care must be exercised in designing phase III clinical trials to ensure that patients to be compared are homogeneous with respect to all known variables, except for the treatment received, thus ensuring their comparability. In addition to patient heterogeneity, physician and patient biases can occur in treatment assignment. For example, physicians might be less inclined to treat debilitated patients with a new drug they perceive to be more toxic than the standard one. Likewise, some patients might refuse a new drug based on anticipated toxicity, personal bias, or other reasons. Alternatively, they might insist on participating in a drug study touted in the mass media to be a *"miracle drug"*, an evocative label often associated with new biotherapeutic agents.

Several study designs have been developed in attempts to reduce patient heterogeneity and drug assignment bias. Of these, *"randomization"* has become the gold standard. As the name suggests, randomization refers to allocating treatment by chance alone without the knowledge of either physician or patient before entering the trial. In practice, each patient eligible for accrual is assigned a given treatment randomly selected by a central computer. The randomization process ensures that each patient has an equal chance of being assigned any of the therapies in the trial, and that the treatment groups will be comparable with respect to factors that might affect the endpoints of the trial, other than the treatment received. Randomization also ensures that, regardless of treatment assigned, all patients are handled uniformly with respect to their management, supportive care, and follow up evaluation while on study. In certain (double-blind) trials, disclosure of the treatment assigned to either patient or physician is not made until completion or termination of the study. After randomized to a treatment group, patients can be further *"stratified"* to subgroups according to well-defined criteria such as age, stage, etc. Benefits of stratification include early detection of side effects, or unusual responses by particular patient subsets but not by the group as a whole. Other important considerations when designing clinical trials include study objectives, choice of end points, eligibility criteria, and sample size, to name but the most important. Many of these are intertwined, thus compounding the degree of difficulty in clinical trial design. For example, a phase III trial in lung cancer will be completed quickly given the modest objectives dictated by the known unresponsiveness of this disease, and a speedy accrual made possible by its high incidence in the population. Alternatively, a trial designed to assess a drug for the treatment of advanced Hodgkin's disease would have to be very large and lengthy given the success of current chemotherapy that yields 80% complete remission rates, with 68% disease-free survival at 10 years [15]. When survival is the main end-point of a trial, off-study treatment of patients who fail to respond or relapse after an initial response might have an impact on outcome that must be considered in the analysis of trial results. This is accomplished by assessing disease-free interval, time to relapse, or time to progression as end-points rather than overall survival.

A most important feature of the modern clinical trial is the use of statistics to determine whether the outcome of a trial, either positive or negative, is likely to be drug-related or a chance occurrence. It is based on the frequency theory of probability that a given outcome of an experiment will be confirmed if sufficient repetitions of the experiment are undertaken. When comparing two drugs or events, two outcomes are possible: the two drugs are equivalent or they differ, also called the null and alternate hypothesis, respectively. Statistical tests enable assessing the level of probability that apparent differences in outcome or lack thereof are erroneously so (α or type I, and β or type II errors, respectively). In practice, a calculated probability above 5% (p value > 0.05) is accepted as evidence that differences in outcome could well be due to chance or experimental variations, whereas a p value < 0.05 infers that the differences, whether positive or negative, are real. Additionally, the level of significance and the magnitude of the expected differences between experimental and control groups will determine the number of patients required in the trial in order to avoid type I or II errors. For example, a drug toxic to 10% of individuals will have a 65% chance of inducing toxicity in at least 1 of 10 patients, but an 89% chance if toxicity affects 20% of individuals. Conversely, in the same example the chances of eliciting at least one toxic episode will rise with sample size, from 65% if 10 individuals are studied, to 96% if 30 subjects are exposed. Thus, the impact of expected differences and sample size on study outcome are pivotal to the design of clinical trials. For example, to confirm with a 90% confidence level, the superiority of a drug with an expected 60% cure rate over an alternate drug with a known 55% cure rate would require accruing 4,100 individuals to the trial, whereas only 112 patients need be enrolled if the cure rate of the alternate drug is only 30% [16]. The likelihood that a positive outcome is truly positive is strengthened by the *"prior probability of success"* (or "θ" factor) for that drug in prior studies. It is tantamount to saying that positive outcomes are more likely that not to be true positive if the drug under study has yielded positive results in prior studies.

Finally, because today's cancer drugs are largely inefficacious, phase III clinical trials often yield no differences between the experimental and standard treatment arms or small differences that are statistically significant but clinically irrelevant [16]. Attempts to magnify such inconclusive results revolve around two strategies. The first is to enroll large numbers of patients in a single trial to increase the discriminant power of the statistical analysis. The second is to use a statistical technique called meta-analysis that analyzes the combined results of several small trials in hopes of uncovering small differences not revealed in individual small trials. However, the latter strategy is invalid when applied to trials that differ in design, therapies, types of patients, quality, or goals. The rationale and relevance of large trials and meta-analysis of small ones is that uncovering small differences in cure rates or survival, especially in cancers with high incidence rates, might save hundreds of lives or benefit thousands of patients each year. Meta-analysis can also lead to unexpected findings counter to the prevailing perceptions. For example, a meta-analysis of all phase III clinical trials conducted in North America between 1973 and 1994 in non-small cell lung cancer revealed that these patients' survival remained unchanged after 2 decades of clinical trials [18]. It is noteworthy that instead of emphasizing this point the author concluded: *"Future phase III trials should be sized appropriately, with at least 200 patients per treatment arm, in order to detect an expected 2-month prolongation of survival between therapeutic regimens"*. The prevailing tendency towards large studies, necessitated by the inefficacy of cytotoxic drugs, is illustrated by the fact that 18 of 101 active phase III trials sponsored by the European Organization for Research and Treatment of Cancer in 2002 were designed to enroll between 1,000 and 4,400 patients each [19]. However, because inefficacious treatments yield negative results large studies are often no more conclusive than small ones as illustrated by the *Tamoxifen for Prevention of Breast Cancer study*, a clinical trial sponsored by the *National Surgical Adjuvant Breast and Bowel Project* and funded by the National Cancer Institute.

This study, which by 1998 had enrolled 13,388 women at a cost of $68 million, reported that compared to placebo Tamoxifen reduced the risk of breast cancer by 49%, but increased the risk of endometrial cancer by 150%, not to mention increased risks of strokes, deep-vein thrombosis, and pulmonary embolism [20]. Understandably, it has been suggested that unless a woman has a Gail index [21] of 5% or greater (that is, a >5% 5-year risk for breast cancer, compared to a risk >1.66% for women entered in the trial), chemoprevention with Tamoxifen should not be considered [22]. Thus, this study, mired in controversy before it was launched, during its execution, and after its conclusions were revealed, and despite its very large size and its high price tag, has failed to provide clear answers to women with increased breast cancer risk who face the daunting task of weighing one potential risk against another. Moreover, two smaller studies, one British [23] the other Italian [24], did not yield a reduction in breast cancer incidence but confirmed the increased risk of endometrial cancer and of vascular events associated with Tamoxifen. A third study, by the International Breast Cancer Interventional Study, is still in the accrual stages. In contrast to the American study, the European and International studies remain blinded and in time might provide a more definitive answer to the benefits and risks of Tamoxifen chemoprevention of breast cancer. In the meantime, *"perhaps the main conclusion is that there are no clear conclusions at this stage"*, as concluded a recent review of the evidence [25]. The emphasis on very large phase III trials involving thousands of patients seems to be gathering momentum as suggested by a *"me-too"* study, called the STAR trial, launched by the NCI in early 1999. With the participation of more than 500 centers across the United States, Puerto Rico, and Canada, the STAR trial is expected to enroll 22,000 postmenopausal women at increased risk of breast cancer to assess whether *"Raloxifene is as effective in reducing the chance of developing breast cancer as tamoxifen has proven to be"*[26].

In conclusion, the design, implementation, and analysis of clinical trials follow well-established guidelines and statistical principles to objectively and accurately assess differences between experimental and control groups despite the complexities inherent to human biology, trial execution, and data analysis. Hence, the lack of progress in cancer therapy is related not to the tools available for assessing the efficacy of cancer drugs but to reliance on non-specific and inherently inefficacious drugs. Resorting to large studies or to meta-analysis of smaller ones in attempts to uncover small differences in drug activity is an implicit acknowledgement of this fact, and a recognition that progress in cancer control will likely continue to be slow and marginally incremental as long as reliance is placed on cytotoxic drugs with no relevance to the cancerous process. Hence, why do most reports on cancer treatment convey a sense of progress?

Chapter 9

PUBLICATIONS: THE FACTS AND NOTHING BUT THE FACTS?

The aim of all medical research is to accrue scientific knowledge to the medical database, and in so doing, provide the foundation for ultimately improving health care. As a special type of medical research, phase III clinical trials are experiments designed to compare, under controlled conditions, the efficacy of two or more interventions directly on human beings. Thus, phase III clinical trials are unique in that their findings have the potential to alter the treatment of a disease, to enable marketing of innovative drugs or devices, and to shape health-care policy, particularly when published in high-profile peer-reviewed journals of wide circulation. Given their potentially far-reaching consequences and the obstacles to repeating a study with controversial or unexpected results, reports of clinical trials must adhere to higher standards than those required from research studies not directly involving humans. In a perfect world, all parties involved in the process would adhere to entirely altruistic principles focused on a common goal, the scientific truth, and be able to pursue that goal resolutely and without interference. However, reality is often shaped by necessity and circumstances. Indeed, a variety of pressures brought to bear on clinical researchers by their employers, sponsors, and publishers, and self-interest, influence the tone and content of most study reports and virtually all press releases.

Articles describing clinical trials must be screened by *"peer-reviewers"* prior to publication. These are experts in the field called upon by editors to ensure that the study described was designed, implemented, analyzed, and reported according to established guidelines, and that the conclusions reached are commensurate with the findings. Peer-reviewers, who usually remain anonymous to authors, provide comments and a priority score that serve as a basis for the journal's editorial board to accept or reject the submission. Reports judged meritorious but lacking in data, analysis, or presentation, are referred back to the author with suggestions for revisions. This process, which takes at least two months to complete, is currently being challenged as a closed system with known deficiencies and biases but no proven benefits [27] that stifles, for profit, the widest and timely dissemination of scientific knowledge [28]. A constellation of reasons, some obvious, some less so, drives medical researchers to publish, one of which is highlighted by the ominous "*publish or perish*". The most obvious and altruistic reason to publish is to disclose results that might serve patients and society, particularly when the benefit is the cure of disease, prolongation of survival or, in their absence, alleviation of suffering. This, in fact, is the primary reason physicians engage in clinical research, along with the personal satisfaction of "*making a difference*" even if that difference is a modest one. However, the world of medical researchers does not evolve in a vacuum, but within society with all its pressures and biases. These pressures and biases take many forms, including career advancement, shifting priorities in research funding, and the increasing link between research productivity and job security, to name only the most important considerations researchers must address in order to survive. For example, at most universities and research centers, salary and career advancement, such as rank promotion and tenure, are formally linked to scientific productivity that is judged by the number of research publications within a certain time frame, and to revenue generation. However, neither addresses scientific merit or social impact. Indeed, a single publication in a high-profile journal is likely to have a greater impact, at least on other scientists if not on society at large, than several articles in second-rated journals. Yet, the same high-profile journal might reject an article addressing a seemingly mundane issue of substantial social impact while publishing another judged of greater scientific value by its reviewers, despite lacking social impact [29]. Moreover, scientific merit and productivity often take a back seat to institutional or programmatic priorities [30] making revenue generation the deciding factor. This is because priorities, at both the national and local levels, change with time in response to political, societal, and economic pressures, not to mention the whims of administrators at many universities and research centers who value medical research solely as a source of revenue. As a result, an increasingly large component of researchers' salaries derives from extramural funds, forcing them to add self-interest to their overall altruistic goal of helping society. In such an environment, researchers must adapt their research interests and direction in order to secure funds for their laboratory and adequate salaries for themselves. In the case of clinical researchers, these multiple pressures might lead to a "*follow the crowd*" mind-set studying the "*drug-du-jour*", either as part of multi-institutional cancer groups mainly supported by NCI, or as *"solo"* investigators funded by pharmaceutical companies in their quest to market a new drug, or to expand the clinical indications for an old one. It is ironic that the lack of progress in cancer management guarantees the survival and continued prosperity of both types of approaches. Indeed, some of the oldest cancer groups, such as the National Surgical Adjuvant Breast and Bowel Project [31] and the Southwest Oncology Group [32] include on their web sites 40-year and 56-year longevity statements, respectively, and the cumulative number of patients accrued to their studies since their inception as implicit indication of success.

Pharmaceutical companies are having an increasing impact on clinical research as highlighted by the fact that in 1999 their combined research and development budget was $22.7 billion whereas the NIH total expenditures were $17.8 billion. Moreover, while NIH expenditure is skewed towards basic science research, the pharmaceutical industry focuses heavily on clinical research, paying $1,000 to $3,000 for each patient enrolled in clinical trials, a lucrative source of revenue for clinical researchers and their employers. However, although drug companies are profitable enterprises, only 5 out of approximately 1,000 drugs reach the clinical trial stage and only 1 receives FDA-approval for patient use. Additionally, only 3 out of 10 marketed drugs generate sufficient revenues to recover the estimated $500 million average research and development costs per drug [33]. Thus, in efforts to control costs, the drug industry often hires non-academic research organizations rather than academic researchers to do the same work at a lower cost, often more expeditiously, and with fewer hassles [34]. That gives drug companies leverage when dealing with cash-poor clinical researchers, often dictating the trial design, sequestering the raw data generated, and allowing little input in data interpretation and conclusions. As a result, published trials supported by the pharmaceutical industry tend to favor the innovative rather than the standard treatment more often than NCI-funded trials [35], and trials with unfavorable outcome might never be published [36]. A 2002 survey of the influence of private industry on clinical trials conducted at 108 participating US medical schools concluded, *"Academic institutions routinely engage in industry-sponsored research that fails to adhere to International Committee of Medical Journal Editors guidelines regarding trial design, access to data, and publication rights. Our findings suggest that a reevaluation of the process of contracting for clinical research is urgently needed"* [37]. Acknowledging conflicts of interest issues of research sponsored by the pharmaceutical industry and the potential harm to society of biased research, published vicariously in the name of academic researchers, editors of 11 leading journals recently announced they will *"routinely require authors to disclose details of their own and their sponsor's role in the study"* [38].

However, the impact of this seemingly bold step is likely to be small given the non-participation of most editors and the fact that such disclosure and data quality are unrelated issues. More on this later.

As for the popular press, reports of medical news are often presented as *"breakthroughs"* in headline or sound- and print-bite formats most favored by the public at large. Alternatively, short interviews are conducted with *"leading scientists"* about recent *"discoveries"* and their potential benefits to humanity. This modus operandus, justified by the *"public's right to know"* the outcome of public funds for medical research, frequently involves an attractive format under evocative names (witness CBS' *"Medicine on the cutting edge"* and ABC's *"Medical File"*) for maximum impact on a receptive public. Interestingly, the origin of most such stories is not the inquisitiveness of journalists but the self-interest of researchers and pharmaceutical companies eager to promote their own agenda. Not surprisingly, most reports of breakthroughs are based on preliminary in vitro or animal studies accompanied by unrealistic future health care projections, years ahead of any potential clinical applications. Understandably, when medical breakthroughs fail to meet expectations follow-up stories are seldom if ever reported, for negative medical news attracts neither audiences nor advertisers. The question of whether media reporting of medical news plays a role in public health depends on whether they capture patients' imagination or influence physicians' practice patterns. While most cancer patients rely on their physician's advice, a substantial number obtain medical information from newspapers (86%) or television and radio (82%) [39], that can lead them to question their physician's judgment or entice them to participate in clinical trials for personal gain. For example, in a recent study 47 of 100 patients who entered a high-profile phase I trial first heard about the trial from media reports, and 77% of them cited hope for personal benefit as the main reason for their willingness to participate [40]. Whether such media reports are misleading or misinterpreted, the fact remains that phase I studies are designed to assess drug toxicity where chances of any personal benefits are near zero; facts seldom mentioned in the news. Despite their potential impact on the public, the content and tone of medical news in the popular press is often shaped by journalists' sketchy scientific background that limits their ability to comprehend and communicate the complexities of modern medical science. For example, an analysis of 306 representative newspaper articles on cancer chosen at random [41] revealed major deficiencies including: misleading titles in 47.5%; no traceable citations (name of journal, researcher, or institution) in 40%; and erroneous information or lack of clarifying data in 55%. Only 13.6% placed the information in the proper context. In an effort to improve journalistic communication to the public of results of medical research and to place each report in the proper context,

NIH recently launched an annual symposium for journalists entitled *"Medicine and the Media: The challenge of reporting on Medical research"*. The symposium was designed to *"prepare participants for the crucial task of evaluating research findings, selecting stories that hold meaningful messages for the public, and placing them in the appropriate context"* [42]. Astonishingly, only 28 participants attended the first symposium, held in June 2002. Finally, a recent and more insidious approach for shaping public perceptions on health issues is the ubiquitous *"ask your doctor"* TV advertisement genre espoused by drug manufacturers to promote sales of new and more expensive drugs. This drug marketing approach risks both threatening the prescribing integrity of physicians and eroding the patient-physician relationship in favor of the pharmaceutical industry's balance sheets. In this context it is not surprising that, helped by well designed advertisements and its undeniable impact on patients well-being, the anti-anemia agent Procrit ® became the 4th best-seller drug in 2003, with 3.3 billion dollars in sales, behind Lipitor ® (6.8 billion), Zocor ® (4.4), and Prevacid ® (4.0). It must be acknowledged that at the other end of the spectrum there are some remarkably well documented and superbly edited medical reports, especially in specialized print and electronic media. However, given their focus on topical health issues of human interest with a happy ending and their limited reach confined to a small segment of the population with a higher level of formal education, the impact of such reports on the public at large is negligible.

In conclusion, clinical cancer researchers, their sponsors, employers, and publishers, and the mass media are motivated by a mixture of altruism, career advancement, notoriety, financial gain, and other incentives. In short, they are human. On the other hand, the vast majority of cancer reports, whether published in the scientific literature or the popular press and regardless of source, are carefully crafted to convey progress. This is because, the parties involved in reporting clinical cancer research, notably medical editors and the mass media, are not interested in negative reports, nor is the public. This creates a spiral of collective optimism about cancer that reinforces the self-delusion of the medical community, and the erroneous perception by policy makers and the public that the *War on Cancer* is on track and the cure of cancer is at hand. Yet, scratching the veneer surface reveals glaring discrepancies between unending optimistic reports and deceiving cancer mortality. As remarked in a widely quoted Lancet editorial about breast cancer [43], *"If one is to believe all the media hype, the triumphalism of the profession in published research, and the almost weekly miracle breakthroughs trumpeted by cancer charities, one might be surprised that women are dying at all from this cancer"*.

Chapter 10

FROM THE DOCTORS' PERSPECTIVE

Thus far, we have shown that clinical cancer researchers and their sponsors, and the scientific and popular press have contributed to creating an atmosphere of optimism regarding cancer that is reinforced by nearly every new report and public announcement. However, given the fact that approximately 98% of all cancer patients are treated by community oncologists outside of clinical trials and both find themselves at the *"receiving end"* of the cancer information chain, we must review their attitudes and perceptions, for they are the final arbiters of patient care.

1. PHYSICIANS' QUALIFICATIONS

1.1 Training and board certification

Oncologists and Hematologists are highly trained Internal Medicine specialists with special expertise in the diagnosis and treatment of malignant diseases. In the US, Hematology was born as a separate medical discipline when 150 physicians met in Boston in April 1958 and formed the American Society of Hematology. It became a sub-specialty of the American Board of Internal Medicine (ABIM) [44] in 1972 when 374 physicians passed the certifying examination and became Diplomates in Hematology. Medical Oncology became a subspecialty of Internal Medicine also in 1972 and the first certifying examination was offered in 1973 with the first 351 Oncology diplomas being issued that year. The ABIM, a private organization that regulates and certifies all Medical specialties in the US, establishes a sequence of qualifications as prerequisites to apply for certification in

Internal Medicine and in all Medical subspecialties. To be awarded a certificate in Internal Medicine *"Physicians must have completed the required pre-doctoral medical education, met the postdoctoral training requirements, demonstrated clinical competence in the care of patients, and passed the Certification Examination in Internal Medicine"*. Pre-doctoral education must have been in an accredited Medical School, and post-graduate training must include *"36 months of graduate medical education accredited by the Accreditation Council for Graduate Medical Education, the Royal College of Physicians and Surgeons of Canada, or the Professional Corporation of Physicians of Quebec. The 36 months of residency training must include (1) a minimum of 12 months of internal medicine training at the R-1 level, and (2) a minimum of 24 months of training in an accredited internal medicine program, 12 months at the R-2 level and 12 months at the R-3 level"*. In addition, candidates must document competence *"in clinical judgment, medical knowledge, clinical skills (medical interviewing, physical examination, and procedural skills), humanistic qualities, professionalism, and provision of medical care"*, and show proficiency in a number of procedures frequently needed in the practice of Internal Medicine.

Only physicians certified in Internal Medicine (185,135 as of April 28, 2003) can apply for certification in a Medical subspecialty such as Medical Oncology or Hematology. To qualify in either subspecialty, physicians are required to take an additional 24 months of specialty clinical training, whereas physicians seeking dual certification in Medical Oncology and Hematology must complete 36 months of additional training. As of April 2003, 9,116 American physicians had been awarded a diploma in Medical Oncology and 5,587 in Hematology, representing 3.2 Oncologists and 2.0 Hematologists per 100,000 persons. A number of these individuals are certified in both, Hematology and Medical Oncology. Both subspecialties have evolved since their inception. At present, Medical Oncology is strongly entrenched in the diagnosis and treatment of cancer, particularly the delivery of cancer chemotherapy. Oncologists have become the focus point for the management of cancer patients, coordinating the input of Radiation and Surgical Oncologists, and of other members of the interdisciplinary cancer treatment team. Likewise, Hematology has evolved from a discipline initially dedicated to benign blood diseases and coagulation disorders, to one that increasingly focuses on transplantation, genetics, and cellular transduction medicine at one end, and merges with Medical Oncology, at the other. In the practice setting, Hematologists, Oncologists, and Hematology-Oncologists manage the vast majority of advanced cancers in the US, and derive most of their income from administering chemotherapy. Given the overlap in training requirements, and the convergence of Oncology and Hematology with regards to cancer diagnosis and treatment, the term

Oncologists will hereafter refer to all physicians whose primary clinical focus is cancer, whether their original training was primarily Oncology, Hematology, or both. Because of their well-organized and strictly supervised training in all aspects of cancer American Oncologists are, at the outset, highly competent physicians superbly qualified to diagnose and treat all types of cancers. Additionally, the vast majority of them update their knowledge database and clinical skills on a regular basis through Continuing Medical Education.

1.2 Continuing Medical Education

Cancer specialists update their knowledge database, as part of an ongoing and even compulsory continuing medical education process, through formal and informal channels. These include oncology journals addressing a broad range of subjects ranging from cancer prevention, to early detection, to treatment; national meetings organized annually by cancer societies offering diverse professional activities ranging from carefully prepared educational sessions to reports of bench and clinical research; and national or regional seminars sharply focused on specific cancer issues. Finally, a substantial number of single- and multi-authored books addressing a wide variety of cancer subjects are published with regularity. The former are usually theme-driven and are usually neither tutorial nor updated, whereas the latter are didactic with periodic updates. Some multi-authored books are part of multi-volume series with a broad range of subjects that are published over many years. Together, these multiple sources of scientific information constitute a bewildering array of never ending reports that address from the broadest of issues to the narrowest of subjects. For example, the current two-volume set edition of the textbook Cancer: Principles and Practice of Oncology, by DeVita and associates, compiles 3,234 pages organized in 65 didactic chapters written by numerous authoritative contributors, and is updated periodically. To complement this solid source of information, there are numerous journals addressing cancer published mostly monthly, 167 of which make available on-line at least part of their content [45]. Of these, the highly respected biweekly Journal of Clinical Oncology alone contributed 4,838 pages to its subscriber's bookshelves in 2,002, mostly of clinical trial reports. Additionally, Oncologists have the opportunity to attend a variety of scientific meetings, seminars, and conferences that range from the highly informative and updated organized by cancer societies, universities, or research centers, to conferences of variable content and quality held locally by oncology groups, often assisted by one or more guest speakers sponsored by the pharmaceutical industry.

One of the cancer societies with the greatest impact to Medical Oncologists is the American Society for Clinical Oncology (ASCO) [46]. ASCO claims more than 19,000 professional members from 100 countries, representing Medical Oncology, Therapeutic Radiology, Surgical Oncology, Pediatric Oncology, Gynecologic Oncology, Urologic Oncology, and Hematology. Its 2002 annual spring meeting attracted nearly 25,000 attendees eager to learn the results of a variety of ongoing clinical cancer trials, directly from the very investigators conducting the trials, and to gage the direction of cancer research. At the 2002 ASCO meeting, nearly 2,000 eclectic reports were chosen for presentation out of the more that 3,000 that competed for the spotlight. Another group with great influence on practicing Oncologists and Hematologists is the American Society of Hematology (ASH) [47]. The ASH currently has over 10,000 members, mostly from the US (81%), Europe (11%), and Asia (6%). Fifty eight percent of ASH members work at academic institutions, 43% are practicing Hematologists-Oncologists, and 24% are clinical investigators. The ASH's annual fall meeting brings together nearly 20,000 scientists, clinicians, and guests to participate in a well-organized program that includes corporate-sponsored symposia, an educational program, and oral or poster presentations (almost 3,500 in 2002), a substantial portion of which address clinical issues and report results of clinical trials. Because of ASCO's and ASH's large constituencies and broad reach, most of the nation's basic science cancer research and clinical trials are reported at one of these societies' meetings. This and the fact that the vast majority of American Oncologists attend at least one of these meetings each year, suggest the enormous influence these societies exert on continuing medical education and on the direction of cancer care.

Finally, the interplay among Oncologists sharing an academic or community practice is a frequent source of exchange of information. Depending on the level and location of practice, this interplay can be informal or take place in one of two more formal settings: case discussions and journal clubs. As the name suggests, case discussions involve selecting individual cases for presentation to the group based on their didactic value or their diagnostic or management difficulty. Typically, case discussions at academic centers are held weekly and are multidisciplinary. They frequently involve Medical, Surgical, and Radiation Oncologists, Pathologists, Cytogeneticists, Flow cytometrists, and other members of the medical team involved in patient care. On the other hand, the purpose of journal clubs is to review recent medical literature. More informal and with the dual purpose of learning and socializing, journal clubs are often held monthly, usually at the home of each group member on a rotational basis. Finally, a variant of the journal club format involves oral presentations, more frequently held in a restaurant setting than at the work place, by remunerated speakers selected and sponsored by pharmaceutical companies based on their experience and familiarity with one or more of the company's drugs. Here too the level of speakers' expertise and the quality and objectivity of the information presented varies greatly. However, by exalting the benefits of the targeted drug and building goodwill towards the manufacturer hosting the meeting, such speakers serve the company's goals more than the audience's needs.

Hence, the evidence shows that if Oncologists have contributed to losing the *War on Cancer*, it is not because of faulty training, lack of expertise, or insufficient knowledge. Their role is rooted in multiple factors that influence their practice directly or indirectly, as we explore below.

2. FACTORS THAT DICTATE CANCER TREATMENT

As described previously, cures are possible in some patients with hematologic malignancies and certain germinal cancers, and a modest prolongation of survival can be achieved in some patients with other types of advanced tumors. Nevertheless, unless medically or psychologically contraindicated, the vast majority of cancer patients receive chemotherapy alone or in combination with surgery or irradiation, often switching from one drug or drug combination to another in futile attempts to influence the course of the disease. In addition to the financial burden imposed on patients and on society ($41 billion in 1995, the most recent year for which there is information) [48], such treatment is associated with human suffering resulting from the multiple and sometimes fatal side effects and complications of the highly toxic cancer drugs. In order to understand the bases of this apparent incongruity we must analyze the perceptions, expectations, and motives of the parties directly involved, and how they are molded by external influences. From the physicians' standpoint, these factors converge on a collective conviction that if cancer is diagnosed, aggressive management must be instituted, an attitude that derives from and is perpetuated by the notion of "*standard of care*". Physicians' attitudes towards cancer are reinforced by patients' strong desire to overcome the dire consequences of cancer left unchecked, although that determination is often based on an incomplete understanding of the benefits and risks of treatment, and an inherent self-preservation instinct that, given the circumstances, is likely to prejudice a rational choice of action.

2.1   The imperatives of "standard of care"

Standard of care is primarily a legal concept that refers to the level of practice that any average, prudent, and reasonable physician would provide under similar circumstances. It must reflect the art (consensus of opinion) and the science (peer-reviewed literature) of medicine. In essence, from a legal standpoint, standard of care is not necessarily the best, most expensive or technologically advanced care available but one that is considered acceptable and adequate under similar circumstances. Thus, any under- or over-utilization of medical care or providing treatment that is inferior to the norm is unacceptable, unethical, and renders the physician guilty of negligence and malpractice. Under these circumstances and notwithstanding physicians' assertions to the contrary, standard of care determines medical practice in the United States. To the Oncologist, standard of care acquires the additional connotation of being the "*best*" treatment modality for a particular cancer. This conceptual evolution is the outcome of the very design of phase III clinical trials where an experimental drug is compared to the standard or "*best*" treatment regimen for the particular cancer under study. Based on clinical trial results, a standard of care is promulgated or implied for every cancer in medical publications, at cancer society meetings, and at national conferences. The perception created is duly reinforced at local seminars by a legion of guest speakers sponsored by the pharmaceutical industry, coordinated and supported by their field representatives, who eagerly provide complementary information praising the product(s) in question. Because negative reports are seldom published, the vast majority of the information conveyed describes "*progress*", "*improvements*", and "*advances*", in cancer management along with the subliminal message that cancer management is choosing between two or more drugs or drug combinations, rather than whether the potential benefits justify the risks. Under these circumstances substantial departures from standard of care practice, including withholding any of the many inefficacious treatments commonly used to manage refractory cancers, could be construed as negligence and malpractice.

When applied to malignancies amenable to cures such as Hodgkin's disease, testicular cancer, and a few other curable cancers (Table VII), standard of care has profound practical and ethical implications. Indeed, in such cases the benefit/risk ratio is dramatically shifted towards benefit thus justifying a relatively high degree of risk to achieve a cure. Ironically, risks associated with curative and non-curative chemotherapy regimens are similar, with the notorious exception of acute leukemia, where a complete ablation of patients' bone marrow, a prerequisite to achieving complete remissions and some cures, contributes to serious complications including death more often than to cures. In contrast, when applied to non-curative treatments that do not prolong survival meaningfully, standard of care essentially means *"the best"* of a group of fundamentally inefficacious therapies, a highly dubious honor. Yet, many cancer drugs and drug combinations shown to be inefficacious over many years remain in use today because, in the absence of better solutions, they are perceived as providing standard of care. For instance, a recent review of two decades of chemotherapy experience in the treatment of advanced non-small cell lung cancer by the Eastern Cooperative Oncology Group (ECOG) reported an average tumor response rate of 25%, a median patient survival of 25 weeks, and a one-year patient survival of 20%, regardless of the drugs or drug combinations used [49]. While these results are not substantially better than those achieved in previous decades [18], the author concluded, *"It is appropriate to offer chemotherapy to all NSCLC patients with advanced disease, a good performance status, and no medical or psychological contraindications to its use"*. Recommendations such as this, made by leading experts in their field especially when published by high-profile medical journals, are uncritically embraced by community and research Oncologists as the standard of care for day-to-day patient management and against which to judge results of future clinical trials.

The attitude and practice of even skeptical Oncologists are shaped by an unending barrage of clinical reports, each describing the superiority of a drug or drug combination over the alternatives for treating each and every cancer. However, given the marginal efficacy of cancer drugs and the heterogeneity of subjects studied, many phase III clinical trials yield results that are statistically valid but clinically irrelevant. This occurs when statistical differences are not accompanied by meaningful improvements in patients' outcome or toxicity. An example of Oncologists' tendency to apply results of the latest clinical trials to their day-to-day practice can be found in the saga of the chemotherapy regimen known by its acronym *"CHOP"* (Cyclophosphamide, Hydroxydoxorubicin, Oncovin, and Prednisone), a drug combination developed in the early 1970s for the treatment of high-risk (aggressive) non-Hodgkin's lymphoma. Although it was proven more efficacious than previous drug combinations, many competing regimens were proposed and tried (the main ones are known by their acronyms COMLA, ESAP, MACOP-B, m-BACOP, PROMACE-CYTABOM, VACOP-B), and most claimed some advantage over CHOP. As is usually the case, many patients were treated with these drug combinations, often with inferior outcomes to those consistently achieved with CHOP. Indeed, in numerous subsequent head-to-head comparisons, CHOP has shown a superior risk/benefit profile than its contenders and for thirty years remained the combination of choice for high-risk non-Hodgkin's lymphoma, with a cure rate approaching 25% (Table VII). More recently, the combination of CHOP with Rituximab, a monoclonal antibody with activity against B-cell lymphomas, has increased the hematologic and cytogenetic response rates and shown a survival advantage at 2 years when compared to CHOP alone. This combination is currently being heralded as the first therapeutic break in 20 years and as the new *"golden standard of care"* for the treatment of aggressive lymphoma [50]. Yet, an editorial accompanying the article [51] cautioned, *"the difference between the survival curves begins to shrink at 2.5 years....it is of concern that more patient treated with CHOP plus rituximab died from infection, cachexia, or cardiac disease"*. Additionally, from time to time Oncologists witness unexpected responses and occasional long-term survivors among patients afflicted by cancers known for their relentless progression regardless of treatment. Such cases and their therapies tend to be more vividly remembered than those who, as expected, succumbed to their disease within the anticipated time frame, tempting the physician to treat comparable future patients similarly. However, making treatment decisions based on anecdotal long-term survivors of usually unresponsive and relentless cancers, particularly when involving substantial risk, is to allow emotions to prevail over good judgment and to unnecessarily expose patients to the risks of cytotoxic chemotherapy in an attempt to recreate a few memorable though unexplained responses.

In essence, through the promotion of treatment regimens that rely on marginally effective drugs advocated by well-regarded experts in trusted publications, and a lack of better alternatives, standard of care has become a self-gratifying and self-perpetuating concept. It encompasses a broad spectrum of treatments, the outcomes of which range from long-term prolongation of survival in a subset of patients afflicted by chemotherapy-sensitive malignancies, to marginal or no benefits but additional morbidity for the majority of patients with refractory cancers.

2.2   Financial incentives or "the chemotherapy concession"

In most medical practices, the outcome of an office visit is a prescription for medications or for laboratory, imaging, or surgical procedures. In most cases, physicians have no financial interest in the pharmacy filling the prescription or in the facilities performing the procedures, thus averting potential conflicts of interest. The influence of financial considerations on physicians' practices is underlined by the very existence of incentive programs implemented by drug companies and health maintenance organizations [52,53], and well documented in reports of over-utilization of services owned by physicians [54,55]. In one study, for example, ownership of radiotherapy facilities lead to 53% more radiotherapy, 42% higher charges, and 18% less consultation time than national averages. In Oncology practice, the profit motive of many therapeutic decisions is obvious, ubiquitous, and hard to escape. This is because chemotherapy is the only commodity sold from doctors' offices [56] accounting for two thirds of the income of Oncologists in private practice [57,58]. This unique medical practice has been named "*The chemotherapy concession*". As could be expected, there are sound practical justifications for such a modus operandus, even if its implementation raises serious ethical issues and often results in practices ranging from questionable to overtly unethical and abusive.

The genesis of the chemotherapy concession was the decision by Oncologists in private practice to combine delivery of cognitive (clinical assessment) and drug delivery services at their offices. This decision was professionally sound given its convenience to themselves and their patients, and its many advantages. The most obvious benefits include the following: stocking all drugs necessary for expeditious patient care; reducing drug delivery errors (medications are prepared and delivered by trusted, specialized nurses); the prescribing Oncologist (or the assigned nurse) is available on site to respond to any drug reaction or other complication; and providing cancer patients a convenient and soothing environment where they can share experiences and support one another. However, the decision was also financially very astute. Indeed, as in the case of pharmacists, Oncologists purchase drugs in bulk, at discount prices, from wholesalers and sell them to patients one by one and at retail prices. Drug price mark-ups, ranging between 10% or 20% to as high as 200%, have been justified by overhead costs, mainly personnel salaries and amortization of chemotherapy facilities. From a strictly business point of view, such a practice is not in itself unethical though the opportunity for financial rewards creates conflicts of interest that can and do influence choices of drugs and practice patterns.

The income of Oncologists in private practice derives from three components [58]: chemotherapy sales and administration (67%); charges for cognitive services (23%); and laboratory tests performed on site (10%). In contrast, academic Oncologists' incomes are based solely on collections from charges for the time-consuming but less lucrative cognitive services: i.e. office visits, consultations, and the like. In academia, profits from drug sales are credited to the hospital pharmacy and receipts from laboratory tests are credited to the hospital laboratory. In addition, the demographics of patients attracted by private and academic Oncology practices have a major financial impact. Patients who patronize Oncology practices pay their full share of their health care costs through insurance or their own funds. In contrast, academic Oncology practices accept and therefore attract indigent and low-income patients seeking health care subsidized by the state or the institution.

institution. Thus, because a large portion of charges at academic centers are non-collectable and some of the rest is lost to unsound accounting practices, collection rates by academic Oncologists can be as low as 20% (20 cents collected for each $1.00 charged), whereas they reach 95% in tightly-run private Oncology practices. As a result of the chemotherapy concession and differences in collection rates, the income of Oncologists in the private sector is on the average two- to three-fold that of their academic colleagues [57,58]. According to the Hospital and Healthcare Compensation Service, the compensation in the year 2000 for Hematologist-Oncologists *"in practice three-plus years"* ranged from $155,475 to $473,000, with an average of $269,298. A comparable mean compensation ($258,404) was reported by the Medical Group Management Association [59]. Well-established Oncologists practicing in large urban areas can gross well in excess of 1 million dollars per year.

Such more than adequate remuneration should deter Oncologists from exploiting the chemotherapy concession for additional financial gain. However, numerous reviews of practice patterns indicate otherwise. Expenditures of outpatient cancer drugs rose from $1,218 per patient in 1995 to $2,003 in 1998, due mostly to a shift towards newer and more costly intravenous drugs [60]. Is the shift justified solely by the beneficial properties of the new agents, or is the profit-motive a consideration? Two recent surveys [61,62] examined this question in the context of the unprecedented acceleration in the use of colony stimulating factors (CSF) after their FDA approval in 1991. Their conclusions were, *"the most important determinant of support for CSF use was being in a fee-for-service practice"* [61], and *"In general, physicians at academic medical centers and in Health Maintenance Organization practices were more likely to prefer dose reduction strategies over addition of CSF, while fee-for-service physicians preferred the opposite strategies"* [62]. While egregious abuses involving disregard for patients' welfare are not rampant, there are countless circumstances and opportunities for engaging in subtle practices that base treatment decisions on financial considerations. Examples include: medically unjustified ancillary treatment, such as using CSF and erythropoietin outside of recommended ASCO indication guidelines [63]; selecting intravenous rather than oral cancer drugs of comparable efficacy, such as VAD (Vincristine, Doxorubicin, and Dexamethasone) rather than oral Melphalan plus Prednisone for multiple myeloma [64]; selection of newer and more profitable but not necessarily more efficacious chemotherapy such as rituximab or rituximab plus CHOP instead of CHOP alone for the treatment of refractory indolent (low-risk) small cell lymphoma [65], which helped propel its 2002 sales to $1 billion [66], five short years after its FDA approval; selection of drug regimens that require frequent office visits, such as COMLA (Cyclophosphamide, Vincristine,

Methotrexate, Leucovorin, and Cytarabine) that requires 11 office visits within 71 days over the more efficacious CHOP which requires one office visit monthly; and embracing highly profitable though unproven cancer management approaches as was the choice of high-dose chemotherapy with stem cell rescue as the preferred treatment for advanced breast cancer [67,68] without any prior studies supporting its benefits. While pressures from patients, patient advocates, and policy makers played crucial roles in the adoption of bone marrow transplants before clinical trials were conducted, private and academic transplanters were quick to oblige. Universities, cancer centers, and private offices scrambled to offer transplanting services, less to improve or complement their existing programs than as an income-generating procedure that eventually proved no better for breast cancer than standard chemotherapy. Another inappropriate choice of drugs can be found in the management of chronic lymphocytic leukemia (CLL). CLL is more often than not a slowly progressive, symptom-free malignancy for which a variety of treatments is available in the clinical setting [69]. They include Chlorambucil with or without Prednisone, COP (Cyclophosphamide, Vincristine, and Prednisone), CHOP, purine analogues (Fludarabine and Cladribine), monoclonal antibodies (Campath-1 and Rituximab), and bone marrow transplantation (autologous and allogeneic) [69]. Of these, Chlorambucil and Fludarabine are the most active agents. The former is an oral, better tolerated, less toxic medication that is less costly and requires fewer office visits than Fludarabine and the other options. Long-term randomized trials and meta-analysis of multiple individual trials have demonstrated that while Fludarabine induced faster and more durable tumor responses than chlorambucil, COP, or CHOP, these improved tumor responses were not translated into prolonged patient survival, in spite of greater toxicity and more complications [70-72]. Nevertheless, flying in the face of the evidence, fludarabine was proposed as *"the drug of choice for the majority of patients with CLL"* [73], a recommendation that has been quickly embraced by the Oncology community propelling sales of fludarabine to over $160 million in 2002 [74]. It must be said that some income-generating practices might be adopted inadvertently, because of information flows or as emulation of practice trends.

William Osler, a renowned Canadian physician and medical historian, reputed to have been the most brilliant and influential teacher of medicine in his day, preached that *"The practice of Medicine is an art, not a trade; a calling, not a business; a calling in which your heart will be exercised equally with your head"* [75]. Little did he know that modern medical practice, particularly Medical Oncology, would bear little resemblance to that ideal in a world where wealth and material possessions are the hallmark of success. However, not withstanding the ethical implications of the chemotherapy concession and the abuses it engenders, perhaps the most questionable practice in Medical Oncology, adhered to by most private and academic Oncologists, is the administration of chemotherapy to patients with advanced cancers historically proven not amenable to cures or survival prolongation. The sequence begins with *"first line"* drugs or drug combinations that historically have elicited the best tumor responses. Patients with unresponsive tumors and those whose cancers relapse after an initial response are then treated with equally inefficacious but equally toxic *"second line"* regimens. Few patients so treated show clinically meaningful responses. In a third phase, most patients are treated with *"salvage"* therapies, a euphemism with little practical meaning. That being the fate of most cancer patients, why do they acquiesce to potentially toxic treatment if the prospects of a cure or survival prolongation are remote? The answer lies in patients' attitudes towards cancer and the grim reality they face.

Chapter 11

FROM THE PATIENTS' PERSPECTIVE

1.   PATIENTS' PERCEPTIONS AND EXPECTATIONS

Facing a diagnosis of cancer can be psychologically devastating. The state of mind of most patients evolves through several phases [76]: denial, then *"why me?"* (crying, anger, and rage), dejection and depression (withdrawal and fear), often followed by a resolute determination to *"fight"* and, towards the end, withdrawal or inner peace and the acceptance of death. Thus, it is not surprising that most patients opt for treatment: any treatment that promises benefits and offers some hope. This forward-looking fighting spirit, anchored on the primeval human instinct of self-preservation, often leads to a selective understanding of information disclosed by the physician; retaining positive elements while rejecting or not registering negative ones. Indeed, even in the US and other Western societies where *"breaking bad news"* has become a largely accepted practice [77,78], patient comprehension of treatment risks and benefits is heavily influenced by diverse factors. These include: the content of the disclosure (thoroughness, clarity, and specificity of the language used); the disclosure venue and timing (hospital, office, and context settings); and the level of personal interest and empathy conveyed by the physician [79]. Conversely, in many regions of the world physicians often censor the information shared with cancer patients in misguided attempts to protect them from the potential emotional or psychological harm of bad news [80-82]. This attempt to shelter patients has the unintended consequence of increasing fear and anxiety, and of depriving them of the empowering feeling conferred by their active participation in the decision-making process

127

and in their own care. In societies where disclosing bad news is accepted practice, patients often control the type and amount of medical information disclosed to them depending on their level of anxiety, ability to cope, and other personal factors. For example, while some patients demand full disclosure in order to actively participate in their own care, patients with the greatest fear of death and a perception of poor prognosis intuitively prefer minimal disclosure, relinquishing all decisions to the physician [83]. In the end, most cancer patients defer to their physicians the choice of therapy, especially when treatment recommendations are presented with conviction. In order to bring into focus the issue of physician-patient communications and to explore their impact on treatment decisions and their legal implications, a clear distinction must be drawn between medical research undertaken within the framework of clinical trials and patient care delivery in the community setting. This is necessary because, as research experiments conducted on human subjects, clinical trials are regulated by Federal laws that require all human research be conducted according to basic ethical principles that ensure respect for the individual, beneficence, and justice, and that participation be informed, voluntary, and not influenced or coerced in any way. In contrast, medical practice in the community setting follows informal standard of care guidelines.

1.1 Disclosure within clinical trials

The first international codification of principles to guide clinical researchers involved in medical research is known as The Declaration of Helsinki. This document entitled *"Ethical Principles for Medical Research Involving Human Subjects"* was adopted by the 18th World Medical Association general assembly meeting in Helsinki, in June 1964. Its 13th principle reads, *"In any research on Human beings, each potential subject must be adequately informed of the aims, methods, sources of funding, any possible conflicts of interest, institutional affiliations of the researcher, the anticipated benefits and potential risks of the study, and the discomfort it might entail. The subject should be informed of the right to abstain from participation in the study or to withdraw consent to participate at any time without reprisal. After ensuring that the subject has understood the information, the physician should then obtain the subject's freely-given informed consent, preferably in writing"*. In the US, codification of human research began when the National Research Act, creating *"the National Commission for the Protection of Human Subjects of Biomedical and Behavioral Research"*, was signed into law on July 12, 1974. Among other tasks, the commission was charged to identify the basic ethical principles that should underlie the conduct of biomedical and behavioral research involving human subjects, and to develop guidelines, which should be followed to assure that such research is conducted in accordance with those principles. The commission first met on February 1976 at the Smithsonian Institution's Belmont Conference Center. Monthly deliberations followed over a period of nearly four years, which resulted in a Department of Health and Human Services' publication entitled: "*The Belmont Report: Ethical principles and guidelines for the protection of human subjects of research*" [84], also known as the Belmont Report for short.

The Belmont Report expanded the Nuremberg Code that had been drafted in 1947 as a set of standards for judging researchers who conducted unethical biomedical experiments on concentration camp prisoners during WWII, and was designed to prevent repetition of medical research abuses revealed in 1972 regarding the natural history of untreated syphilis. This referred to a study conducted in the 1940's on 399 poor black males from Tuskegee, Alabama who were not informed of their disease and denied penicillin when it became available in 1947, leading to a full enquiry and an apology by President Clinton in 1997 [85]. Other infamous unethical experiments, highly implausible today thanks to legislation enacted since, came to light in a 1993 exposé by *The Albuquerque Tribune*. It revealed both the injection of radioactive tracers to thousands of unsuspecting human subjects, and the radiation exposure of thousands of unaware individuals to several hundred secret and intentional releases of radiation over a 30-year period. As a result, on January 15, 1994 President Clinton created the Advisory Committee on Human Radiation Experiments to investigate reports of unethical conduct of the US government and of institutions funded by the government, in the use of, or exposure to, ionizing radiation in human beings during the period 1944 through 1974. In its final report [86], the panel described the following illustrative case. Mr. Cade, a fifty-three-year-old "*well developed and well nourished colored male in good health*", was hospitalized at the Oak Ridge Army hospital on March 24, 1945 for arm and leg fractures resulting from an auto accident. On April 10th, Mr. Cade, now identified as "HP-12" (HP was the code name for "human product"), was injected with 4.7 micrograms of plutonium without his consent and blood and bodily excretions were tested for radioactivity at several intervals. Five days later his broken bones were set and sampled for radioactivity. More egregiously, identified as having "*marked*" tooth decay, fifteen of his teeth were extracted and tested for plutonium.

From the Belmont Report and subsequent legislative efforts was born the modern Informed consent, a document that discloses in detail: I) the title, purpose, type, design, duration, risks and benefits of the study; II) alternative treatment options under consideration; III) confidentiality and patient rights issues; and IV) independent sources where patients can obtain additional information. The participating subject must sign it after having had an opportunity to discuss and clarify issues of concern with the study's principal investigator. The oversight and responsibility for implementation of these guidelines rest with the Institutional Review Boards [84] at institutions where human research is conducted. The informed consent also brings uniformity to the disclosure process, engages patients' participation in their own treatment, and sets the stage for open and transparent communications between patient and physician.

While in principle the Belmont Report affords a high level of protection to Americans participating in biomedical and behavioral sciences, it was criticized for not addressing social or mind control experimentation [87,88]. More importantly, the Belmont Report and the Informed consent protect the approximately 2% of the total US cancer population who participate in clinical trials at any given time. However, they do not apply to the remaining 98% who receive non-investigational cancer treatment by Oncologists in the community setting. Another loophole is the definition of clinical research, which is often ambiguous and difficult to distinguish from what constitutes small deviations from standard practice. Such deviations are frequent in cancer management because many if not most Oncologists use cancer drugs "*off-label*", that is for indications other than those approved by the FDA or in combinations not sanctioned by prior clinical research, especially to treat patients who have failed standard treatment. This practice is permitted by the definition of "*practice*" in the Belmont report: "*interventions that are designed solely to enhance the well-being of an individual patient or client and that have a reasonable expectation of success*". In contrast, research is defined as "*an activity designed to test a hypothesis... described in a formal protocol that sets forth an objective and a set of procedures designed to reach that objective.*" Although the use of cancer drugs off-label might be justified occasionally by the breath of knowledge and expertise of seasoned Oncologists, the practice is widespread and often based on anecdotal personal experience rather than on clinical trials data. As a result, while unsuspecting patients so treated are exposed to additional and often unforeseen side effects and complications, they seldom benefit.

The quality of the disclosure, or lack thereof, can also be at issue. Indeed, while most Oncologists are conscientious and dedicated to their patients' welfare, the desire to communicate in simple language and time constraints often leads to insufficient disclosure. Alternatively, the zeal for thoroughness might result in disclosure of superfluous and confusing details, or the use of an overly complicated language not readily comprehensible by some patients. Indeed, audio- or video-taped surveys of Oncologists' interviews with prospective clinical trial participants have shown multiple deficiencies in the disclosure process that, in some cases, rendered the Informed consent null and void [87,88]. However, more troubling though less frequent is non-compliance by some unscrupulous or "*market-driven*" researchers who disregard ethical principles and violate Federal rules designed to protect research subjects for expediency or self-serving motives, putting patients at risk and exposing themselves to FDA censure [91], loss of Federal research funding and academic standing [91,92], dismissal [93], or to lawsuits [94]. More ominously, each new revelation of unethical conduct by medical researchers rekindles public distrust in clinical research and raises questions as to whether they represent isolated cases or the tip of an iceberg of misconduct.

1.2 Disclosure in the community setting

It is stating the obvious to assert that the Oncologist planning treatment and the cancer patient being advising should both be aware of the risks and benefits of the recommended treatment and have a clear understanding of the potential outcome. Thus, it might be expected that a substantial number of patients afflicted by advanced cancers of the types proven over the years to follow a relentless course unaffected by chemotherapy would not be offered treatment or decline it if offered. However, the vast majority of cancer patients are treated despite the facts that fewer than 2% achieve a cure and prolongation of survival is the exception as previously described. This is due not only to Oncologists' pro-treatment stance, but also to patients' attitudes regarding cancer treatment. Indeed, studies have shown that patients are willing to accept substantial risks when facing cancer and imminent death. For example, in one study [95] 53.1% of cancer patients expressed willingness to suffer "*severe*" treatment side effects in order to reach a 1% cure rate, 42.1% to survive an additional 3 months, and 42,6% to achieve symptom relief, compared to 20%, 10.2%, and 6.8% of Oncologists, 13.5%, 6.0%, and 5.9% of Oncology nurses, and 19%, 10%, and 10% of healthy controls. Is this risk-taking by cancer patients a rational, weighted decision? Is it the result of over-enthusiastic physicians emphasizing small benefits while minimizing risks? Or, is it the result of unsound decisions driven by the extraordinary stress of individuals confronting cancer and imminent death? In most instances, patients' role in the decision making process is limited to acquiescing to the physician's choice of action after asking but a few questions usually without seeking information from independent sources [96], despite surveys that indicate that most patients in all age groups professes to prefer active participation in decision-making [97]. Indeed, not only do the psychological and emotional impacts of a cancer diagnosis diminish patients' analytical mental power and discerning capacity when it is most needed, but most patients have no desire and make no attempts to independently research their disease or treatment options. Given the circumstances, the instinct of self-preservation usually prevails, leading most patients to hear want they want to hear [98], particularly if the content, setting, and empathy of the disclosure process is sub-optimal.

Trust in the physician is an essential element of the patient-physician relationship. However, a physician becomes a perfect agent for the patient only when the latter would make the same decision if in possession of the same clinical information and expertise. Such a circumstance rarely exists in practice for few patients will achieve a level of understanding comparable to that of their physician and most physicians fail to elicit patients' preferences [99]. In practice, the Oncologist-patient encounters will be multiple over the course of the disease and each time involve three stages, including exchange of information, discussion, and decision-making. The type of interaction depends on the patient-physician relationship that generally takes one of three forms [100]: the traditional "*paternalistic*" model, where information flows in one direction: from physician to patient. The physician makes all decisions regarding treatment and patient management and the patient acquiesces to professional authority and expertise. At the other extreme lies the "*informed*" model where information flows from physician to patient but the patient makes all decisions. Between these extremes is the "*shared*" model where exchange of information proceeds both ways: the physician thoroughly informs the patient of treatment options along with their risks and benefits, and the patient voices preferences, and both contribute to the decision-making process. While by virtue of their training and expertise and for expediency most physicians tend to adopt the paternalistic approach, patients' preferences vary according to age, sex, educational level, and type and severity of the disease. For example, a study of 1,012 women with breast cancer revealed that 22% wanted to select their own treatment, 44% elected to share the task with their physician, and 34% preferred to delegate the responsibility to their physician [101]. Additionally, many patients are receptive to substantial amounts of information, even if they do not wish to participate in making treatment decisions. Under the shared model, patients must be in possession of substantial clinical information in order to participate in treatment decisions that will profoundly affect their lives and often determine their survival. Yet, the physician disclosure process is often inadequate, not geared to patients' needs, and often misleads patients to overestimate benefits and underestimate risks [102]. In attempts to improve the thoroughness and quality of the information transferred from physicians to patients, decision aids in the form of written, audio, video, or computer-based materials have been devised for various cancers [103]. These seldom used aids are valuable mostly to patients who chose the shared model for treatment decisions.

Treatment of cancers historically shown to progress relentlessly regardless of treatment is encouraged by the widespread practice of assessing treatment efficacy by tumor rather than by patient outcomes. Recognizing this general practice, the ASCO recommended that potential benefits of cancer treatment in the clinical setting should be measured, not by tumor outcomes but by patient outcome end-points, including mean or median survival, percent of patients surviving 1, 2, or more years after diagnosis. This information, readily available from the medical literature for all cancers in all stages, should be used as the sole guide for deciding whether or not chemotherapy will be of benefit to a particular patient, and so inform the patient. Tumor outcomes, such as response rates, remissions, and the like, can be discussed. However, physicians must inform patients that the latter represent not goals in themselves but interim assessments of tumor size that are useful to determine whether the therapy instituted is efficacious and worth pursuing or inefficacious and should be abandoned. Physicians should stress that tumor responses have little relevance to the ultimate course of the disease or patient survival. Likewise, potential complications, especially life-threatening toxicity of the treatment contemplated, and their management, should be disclosed at the outset. Alternative treatments, including withholding or delaying treatment, and the effect of each on survival, should be discussed. Likewise, because pain is one of the most feared complications of cancer, patients must be reassured that pain control is easy to achieve in most circumstances given today's potent analgesics. Finally, patients should be encouraged to ask questions, to discuss their options with loved-ones or seek second opinions, and be allowed time for reflection. Oncologists who adopt this advisory role are rewarded by enlightened patients who tend to become participants in their own care, and who have a greater appreciation of the highly complex issues involved in cancer management and, having understood and accepted the risks involved, are less likely to resort to legal action when not warranted.

A written informed consent form patterned after the one familiar to clinical investigators [104] could record all the information described above. However, the expanded form would prominently display the following: 1) a short text or tabular description of the patient's cancer type and stage; 2) the best drug or drug combination for the particular case (cancer type, stage, etc), plus one or two alternative treatment options, each stratified according to their expected patient outcome benefits; 3) the risks associated with each treatment option, stratified by severity and probability of occurrence; 4) disclosure of financial interest in the study, confidentiality, and rights, and; 5) independent sources of medical information pertinent to the case. Such expanded informed consent forms could be developed for each of the more than 200 cancer types, beginning with the 10 most lethal cancers in

American men and women that will account for 70% of all cancer deaths (Figure 1b) projected for 2003 [105]. The task of designing such expanded consent forms could be assigned to panels of experts from NCI, ASCO, ASH, cancer cooperative groups, universities, or research centers and, after securing input and approval by the Medical Oncology community, be made available on the Web not only to physicians but to anyone interested. Some will argue, correctly, that such a document cannot apply to all situations. However, sufficient flexibility can be built in the document to allow modifications according to individual variations in cancer and clinical profiles, with the added advantage that each would be discussed with the patient and recorded as rationale for the selected treatment and for any adjustment contemplated. There is precedent for this in clinical trial protocols where initial and subsequent adjustments to the treatment proposed are allowed in order to individualize care and reduce risks. Moreover, the proposed expansion of the information disclosure process and of the informed consent form would codify, organize, and bring uniformity, transparency, and objectivity to a process that many community Oncologists follow in principle, but in an inconsistent and undocumented manner. Additionally, a thorough, transparent, and objective initial disclosure would serve as a basis for future physician-patient communications and facilitate subsequent management decisions that become necessary during the course of the disease. This approach is applicable to all cancer patients; even those who choose a strictly paternalistic physician-patient relationship model and prefer to be in possession of rudimentary rather than detailed information about their disease and its treatment. In such cases, the information could be conveyed primarily to the next of kin or guardian.

2.   FACING HARD CHOICES

As reviewed in chapter 7, approximately 2% of patients with disseminated or metastatic cancer treated with chemotherapy will be cured of their disease and prolongation of survival is not feasible for most patients afflicted by most types of cancer. Consequently, treating most patients unless contraindicated, as is the practice today, would seem a futile exercise. However, in addition to these most desirable "*quantitative*" patient outcomes, potential "*qualitative*" outcomes, such as objective symptom relief or subjective improvement might justify treatment, including its potential complications and side effects. Indeed, if cure or prolongation of survival is not possible, palliation becomes the Oncologist's major goal. While the above statement is intuitively obvious and unassailable, it embodies concepts that, given their ethical, social, and legal context, are difficult to define and to apply in the clinical arena. For example: What is palliation? Can we distinguish and quantify the placebo component of palliative chemotherapy? When is a cancer judged refractory? When is a treatment futile?

2.1 When to withhold or withdraw treatment

If a cancer patient is unlikely to be cured or survive longer as a result of treatment, is the treatment justified to improve quality of life (QOL)? As previously discussed, the intuitively obvious concept of QOL is neither definable nor quantifiable with any degree of consensus. More ominously, the closely related notion of palliation has two widely divergent and incompatible interpretations in the practice setting: one that properly views palliation in the context of symptom relief; the other that equates palliation with the administration of non-curative treatment presumably aimed at preventing future complications of progressive cancer. While the former addresses patients' immediate QOL needs, the latter justifies inflicting additional pain and suffering now in exchange for a promise of a better future QOL that might or might not be achieved. Thus, given the vagaries of the concept of QOL and the flexible interpretation of what constitutes palliation in the clinical setting context, the present discussion will address the concept of "*futile*" chemotherapy and its subservience to the notion of cancer "*refractoriness*", and the relevance of both to cancer management.

A search for "*medical futility*" literature through Medline yielded 1,057 entries in the last 10 years (August 1992 and August 2002). This high level of interest was stimulated by reports in the late 1980s of patients and their relatives demanding life-sustaining measures judged by their physicians to be futile [106,107]. Such demands, based on a misinterpretation or misuse of the principle of patients' "*rights of autonomy*", are neither legally nor ethically defensible. This is because the rights of autonomy, well established in law and ethics, are negative rights, not positive ones. That is, patients have the right to choose among treatment options offered by physicians, including refusing all treatment despite negative consequences to themselves. However, patients have no right to demand a treatment of their choice not contemplated by their physician, for it would violate physicians' professional integrity. In contrast, the debate and controversy centers on whether physicians can withhold or withdraw a treatment judged "futile", and when can they do so legally and ethically. Resolution of these questions is directly linked to the definition of "medical futility". The term futile derives from the Latin "*futilis*" or leaky, an idea apparently rooted in Greek mythology that through compelling imagery illustrates the two main inherent attributes of a futile endeavor: pointlessness and endlessness. According to this mythical version [108], king Danaus of Egypt had 50 daughters and his brother

Aegyptus had 50 sons. The latter demanded that his sons marry their cousins, an idea vehemently opposed by Danaus. On the wedding day, Danaus instructed his daughters to kill their husbands in the wedding bed. All complied but Hypermnestra who defended her disobedience claiming she remained a virgin after the wedding night. According to legend, the 49 daughters guilty of murder were punished in the underworld by having to continually fetch water carried in sieves.

As a complex concept that incorporates medical, social, ethical, and legal components medical futility has escaped precise definition. In its 1999 *"Code of Medical Ethics"*, the American Medical Association declared, *"medical futility cannot be meaningfully defined"* [109]. However, it is generally agreed that quantitative and qualitative components, also referred to as *"odds"* and *"ends"* [110], should be part of any definition, though there is no consensus on what thresholds should be applied. According to this view, a futile treatment is one that has low probabilities (the *"odds"*) of achieving a desired goal (the *"ends"*). Arguments offered by pro-futility advocates include professional integrity that asserts that physicians should not be required to offer useless or harmful treatments, professional expertise that views the physician as the sole arbiter of treatment selection, and stewardship of scarce resources to be used for beneficial purposes. Critics have raised major concerns. They include, physicians have no grounds to impose their personal values regarding what *ends* can be pursued and at what *odds* [110,111], especially because no consensus has been reached about its definition or application in the clinical setting, clinical trial data are not necessarily applicable to individual patients and, evidence-based outcome standards are lacking in most medical fields. However, while conceptually defensible, critics' arguments become somewhat tenuous in the context of Oncology practice. First, under the informed consent guidelines discussed above treatment decisions are based on a thorough discussion of the pros and cons of available options without pressures from either party. Second, the benefits and risks of cancer treatment are spelled-out in a plethora of clinical trial reports that disclose the anti-tumor activity and untoward effects of cancer drugs in innumerable combinations and permutations for most cancers and in a variety of circumstances. Consequently, in Oncology *odds* and *ends* are well-defined and generally quantifiable entities, except for symptom palliation and QOL that are often used as substitute *ends* in order to rationalize the administration of inefficacious cancer drugs.

A most restrictive definition of medical futility puts the quantitative threshold for *odds* at less than 0.01 (<1%). That is, it considers futile any treatment with less than 1 in 100 chance of benefiting the patient [112]. This definition of medical futility has been criticized on the grounds that it cannot be defined or applied to a given patient; amounts to a usurpation of patients' autonomy, and undermines free exercise of religion. However, its major flaw is its failure to take "*burden*" into account. That is, the physical, emotional, financial, or social costs associated with treatment: the concept of proportionality. However, futility and burden, terms grounded on the ethical principles of beneficence and non-maleficence, are not to be confused. Indeed, a treatment is futile when it does not help (negative beneficence), and burdensome when it causes harm (positive maleficence). While harm is easily detectable and quantifiable, medical futility has a physiological component and a normative one. The former refers to the purpose of the treatment while the later relates to the perception of benefit by physician or patient. As such, it falls in the subjective realm of QOL. Thus, in practice harmful side effects, lack of a tumor response, or less frequently a poor use of resources are the main reasons invoked to withdraw a treatment [113].

Nevertheless, medical futility in Oncology is a special case, for the clinical objectives of cytotoxic chemotherapy are tumor-centered rather than patient-oriented where beneficence is generally judged as a function of tumor-size reduction, and maleficence (harm) to many is implicitly justified by prolonged survival of a few. Is it ethical to risk harming many individuals in order to benefit a few? This issue is particularly pertinent to Oncology where drug toxicity and treatment complications can reach life-threatening severity, including bone marrow, heart, kidney, and lung failure, and fatal infections or bleeding, while objective benefits are modest or nil for most cancer patients. Perhaps the best illustration of lack of proportionality between desired *ends* and *burden* to patients and society has been the relentless dose escalation of a variety of drug combinations for metastatic breast cancer, leading to high-dose chemotherapy with bone marrow rescue. A recently published analysis of several metastatic breast cancer studies representing 30-years of clinical trials demonstrated little difference in overall survival (median of 2 years), whether patients were given standard-dose chemotherapy, high-dose chemotherapy, or high-dose chemotherapy with bone marrow rescue [114]. The latter group included some long-term survivors and, not surprising, some early deaths as well. While sobering in themselves, these conclusions are the more humbling when considered in light of a 1980 study [115] that reported a comparable 2-year overall survival in women with metastatic breast cancer before the chemotherapy era that remained unchanged during the early years of standard chemotherapy. These studies clearly demonstrate that compared to standard-dose treatment, high-dose chemotherapy of breast cancer with or without stem cells rescue, is medically futile for it increases the *burden* to patients (physical, emotional, and financial) and society (misallocation of resources), without clear benefits to most patients notwithstanding an occasional, "*outlying*" long-term survivor.

2.2   Managing patients with refractory cancers

Moralists and bio-ethicists tend to have a perspective of futility that is based primarily on abstract conceptions. In contrast, physicians who frequently face many life and death situations throughout their careers have the experience necessary to steer the debate towards a realistic and practical definition of medical futility, and to guide the development of sensible guidelines for its application in the clinical setting. Oncologists view cancer as an enemy that must be defeated, accounting perhaps for their obstinate determination in pursuing treatment while hope persists, and for considering cures and long-term survivors as personal victories. However, most advanced cancers progress relentlessly regardless of treatment and patients inevitably reach a point of no return, when it becomes obvious to both patient and physician that the end is near and further cancer treatment would be of no benefit and is therefore futile. In most such cases, treatment modalities have been exhausted or chemotherapy tolerance has been reached or breached. It is usually at this late juncture that further cancer treatment is judged futile and the focus becomes symptom relief, ordinarily in the hospice setting. The psychological and emotional impact of reaching that juncture can be reduced by a pre-existing, transparent, and proactive style of physician-patient relationship that will have prepared patients to anticipate, discuss, and accept the inevitable outcome. However, if such an outcome is inevitable for most non-hematologic and non-embryonal malignancies, the question is whether chemotherapy for such cancers is futile from the outset, particularly given the potential harm associated with the relentless administration of inefficacious but toxic treatments.

This question is particularly relevant to the pursuit of high-dose chemotherapy and other strategies attempted over the last thirty years to enhance cancer drug efficacy given their non-specificity. Were the tens of thousands of women with metastatic breast cancer benefited by high-dose chemotherapy, or were they subjected to unnecessary toxicity? It is now clear that instead of relentlessly exploring every conceivable combination of inefficacious drugs in ever escalating doses in search of an elusive efficacious cancer treatment, and devising strategies designed to counteract lethal toxicity, the medical community should have paused and objectively analyzed outcome trends. Instead, a stream of self-serving reports announcing breakthroughs, improvements, and advances appeared in the medical literature and the lay press supporting the status quo. Regrettably, facing reality is often postponed especially when reality contradicts preconceptions and practice patterns. Perhaps this explains why reports of near stagnating survival rates in patients with advanced lung cancer between 1973 and 1994 [18] and metastatic breast cancer between 1980 and 2002 [112] have been all but ignored. Indeed, patients afflicted by these and other chemotherpy-unresponsive cancers continue to be treated with cytotoxic drugs, albeit in new combinations and permutations, with little expectations of improved survival. Hence, in view of these findings should all cytotoxic chemotherapy be considered futile in the context of curing or prolonging survival of patients with historically refractory malignancies and be used as palliative agents instead? This issue is examined below in the context of palliative care.

The debate over medical futility in the US has had the salutary effect of highlighting the notion that a peaceful and dignified death, defined as the natural outcome of aging or the inevitable sequel of a terminal illness that can be eased by end-of-life palliative care, is also a desirable goal. When curative intent or prolongation of survival are no longer feasible the emphasis shifts from disease- to symptom-control focusing on physical, emotional, and spiritual comfort to patients and their families rather than on an obstinate confidence in the unrealistic curative powers of modern medicine. The social and family foundation of the palliative care concept was forcefully articulated by Joseph Califano, former secretary (1977-1979) of the US Department of Health, Education, and Welfare, *"It is time we recognize, in the dependency of the terminally ill, the dignity and beauty of dependency that we long celebrated in the early days of newborn babies. Those with irreversible illness deserve the same loving care as they leave this world that we provide the helpless infants as they enter it"* [116]. This age-old concept, ingrained in most cultures but forsaken in modern societies, has evolved into the *"Hospice"* movement.

The term Hospice derives from the Latin Hospis, which means both host and guest, and hospitium, which refers to the dwelling where guests are greeted with hospitality. While hospitality to pilgrims and traveling strangers was offered from pagan antiquity to the Islamic world, it flourished during the times of the Christian crusades and pilgrimages. During that time hospitiums were found mostly in monasteries where monks assisted the hungry and weary on their way to the Holy Land, Rome, or other holy places, but also extended care to the sick and dying, the woman in labor, the needy poor, the orphan, and the leper on their journey through life. St. Bernard hospice in Switzerland, founded by St. Bernard of Menthon in 962, is the most famous and enduring as it still shelters gratuitously over 20,000 mountain climbers and travelers every year. The practice became especially widespread during the middle ages. For example, the four main pilgrimage routes in France (from Paris, Vézelay, Le Puy, and Arles) to Santiago de Compostela in Spain, each fed by numerous subsidiary routes, spanned over 3,000 miles of roads dotted by over 800 hospitiums or hostels along the way [118]. Millions of pilgrims found shelter and lodging there between the early

XIIth century and the end of the XVIIIth. Many of these hospitiums still offer modern-day pilgrims rest, refuge from the elements, and bed-and-breakfast. The concept of shelter, food, and comfort for the traveling needy was expanded to local populations in 1633 when a French priest, St. Vincent de Paul, founded the Sisters of Charity in Paris. The Sisters' vows were to shelter and care for orphans, the poor, the sick, and the dying. Their success inspired Baron von Stein of Prussia a century later to open Kaiserswerth, the first Protestant hospice, also staffed by nuns. By 1789, the Sisters of Charity operated 426 shelters in France, and many more throughout Western Europe. However, historians and commentators generally credit Jeanne Garnier of France, the Irish Sisters of Charity in Dublin, Ireland, and Cicely Saunders of Britain for evolving the concept of hospice and promoting its worldwide adoption: Jeanne Garnier for opening the first hospice for dying cancer patients in Lyons, France, in 1842; the Irish Sisters of Charity for associating the concept of Hospice to end-of-life care at their Our Lady's Hospice opened in 1879; and Cicely Saunders, of Britain, for emphasizing the psychosocial dimensions to death and dying at Saint Christopher's, the hospice she founded in 1967, and for inspiring followers throughout the world [116].

In the US, the first hospice was opened in 1974. However, the palliative care movement failed to gain momentum mainly due to the enthusiastic and uncritical over-reliance on scientific advances to address purely medical issues while neglecting their psychosocial dimensions. However, two developments led to the recognition of the merits and adoption of the hospice concept by medical organizations, government, and society at large. They include the failure of physicians to provide adequate pain control to terminally ill patients, to acquiesce to their patients' end-of-life care preferences, or ignore them altogether [119], and the convergence of critics of the right to physician-assisted suicide onto the opposing notion of *"physician-assisted living"* [114]. In 1990, the World Health Organization defined palliative care as *"the active total care of patients whose disease is not responsive to curative treatment. Control of pain, of other symptoms, and of psychological, social, and spiritual support is paramount. The goal of palliative care is the achievement of the best quality of life for patients and their families"* [120]. In essence, palliative care in the hospice setting assists preparing for and managing self-determined life closure, the dying process, and death. In the US, adoption and implementation of palliative care remains marginal. For example, in 1983 the Hospice Medicare plan was launched to reimburse care for terminally ill patients (certified by a physician as having six months or less to live). Yet, out of the $210 billion spent by Medicare in 1998, only $2.1 billion (1%) was Medicare hospice care costs despite the fact that six of the ten most costly diseases covered were cancers (lung, prostate, breast, colorectal, pancreas, and recto-sigmoid). Under-utilization of hospice care for the terminally ill in the US is also illustrated by contrasting Medicare hospice costs (1% of total Medicare expenditures) to Medicare payments for hospitalizations and high-tech interventions during the last year of life (28% of total), half of it in the last two months. These statistics strongly suggest that medical care received by Medicare recipients in their last year of life was glaringly inefficacious and therefore futile, despite its high cost. Because palliative care generally does not begin until standard medical care ceases, it is safe to assume that unnecessary additional pain and suffering was inflicted on many of these terminally ill patients. Experience shows that this attitude is prevalent in Oncology where physicians tend to battle cancer beyond the point of no return, inflicting additional burden to patients for little of no gain, neglecting in the process to address patients' psychological, emotional, spiritual, and social needs until the very end.

In conclusion, a rational balance between curative and palliative intent in cancer treatment calls for attitudinal changes by cancer care providers and insurers. Oncologists must focus on patient-outcomes rather than tumor-outcomes, recognize the limitations of cytotoxic drugs in curing cancer or prolonging survival, identify the most propitious time to forgo chemotherapy in favor of standard non-cytotoxic palliative care measures. They should also devote as much effort and enthusiasm in providing comprehensive palliative care to terminally ill patients and their families, as they display when aggressively treating newly diagnosed cancer. Likewise, third party payers must fully embrace the hospice concept as a humane and cost-effective approach to the palliative care of the terminally ill, and lift current restrictions to access and limitations in coverage. While these measures are essential to provide adequate and dignified end-of-life care, a paradigm shift will be necessary to lift cancer management out of its lethargy. The bases for the new model are two-fold. First, the acknowledgement that the cell-kill paradigm and the drugs it fosters to wage War on Cancer have not produced the desired results despite the enormous expenditures in terms of human and financial resources spent over several decades. Second, adoption of a fundamentally different, evidence-driven model capable of curbing both the incidence and mortality of cancer, and eventually add this disease to the list of controllable chronic human ailments.

PART V

WHERE DO WE GO FROM HERE ?

Chapter 12

A VISION FOR THE FUTURE

Predicting the next revolution in cancer care is admittedly an uncertain undertaking but cumulative evidence of a system gone astray and nascent trends for correction are unmistakable. Until recently, researchers and their sponsors focused their efforts, and clinicians and their patients centered their hope more on the eradication of advanced cancer than on its prevention or detection in surgically curable early stages. This arose from the belief that cancer represents a seldom preventable, deadly tissue growth that is difficult to diagnose in early stages, is distinct from the host and, as such, must be eradicated. However, while surgery is adept at eradicating early-stage cancer, the types of cancer drugs fostered by the notion of non-self are inefficacious in altering patients' outcome, and the notion itself was proven obsolete by recent advances in cancer genetics. Additionally, it is increasingly clear that translational application of cancer genetics data is the foundation for the emerging pharmacogenomics of the future that will replace the trial-and-error approach of the past. Thus, the time has come to develop a new approach to cancer control based not on eradication at any cost but on comprehensive, stepwise, and evidence-based measures. They include prevention, early diagnosis, and, when these fail, on controlling the aberrant molecular genetic pathways underlying the development, growth, and dissemination of cancer (the caveat *"when these fail"* underscores the difficulties of controlling complex genetic abnormalities often associated with advanced cancer). Adoption of such broad-based cancer control measures requires a fundamental paradigm shift [1] of such a magnitude and reach that its adoption and implementation is likely to be resisted by supporters of the old, cell-kill paradigm. Indeed, as Max Planck the physicist who postulated the quantum theory observed, *"An important scientific innovation rarely makes its way by gradually winning over and converting its opponents ... Instead, opponents gradually die out and the new generation adopts the idea from the beginning"*. It might be argued that old hypotheses about the nature of cancer and theories about its treatment seemed cogent when first proposed and were proven wrong only in retrospect, and that the new paradigm might also lead us adrift. However, the inability of the old paradigm to explain most of the recent scientific tenets regarding the nature of cancer and its inadequacy as a foundation for spawning efficacious treatments can be neither redeemed, redressed, nor improved by any future discoveries potentially on its path. In contrast, the new paradigm is anchored on new scientific information regarding the nature, development, and progression of cancer and is supported by clinical studies that provide proof of concept of each of its component parts. Indeed, the crucial role played by prevention and screening on declining of cancer incidence rates recorded since 1992 was underscored in NCI's 2001 Cancer Progress Report [2]. It acknowledged, *"Behind the numbers are declines in certain behaviors that cause cancer, especially cigarette smoking by adults. More people are getting screened for breast, cervical, and colorectal cancers"*. Likewise, the success of Imatinib mesylate, a drug developed to harness the molecular defect that causes chronic myelocytic leukemia rather than to kill the leukemic cells, and its success in the clinical arena provide proof of concept in support of molecularly targeted agents of the future. Thus, because it is sound in conception, based on scientific and clinical evidence, and of plausible implementation, the proposed new paradigm is likely to succeed in controlling cancer. Nevertheless, cognizant of the enormity of the task at hand and of the difficulties lying ahead my purpose is not to impose my vision for the future but to encourage a long overdue paradigm shift that is necessary to ultimately control cancer, whether or not it follows my proposal. The fate of over one million Americans who develop cancer each year, and millions more around the World, depend on it.

1.   CANCER PREVENTION

For a cancer prevention program to be successful, it must fulfill three fundamental requirements. First, it must be evidence-based: i.e. be based on a well-established causal-effect relationship between cancer and carcinogens or cancer-promoting habits to be avoided. Second, it must set achievable goals, i.e. recognize that success will hinge upon the combined and sustained cooperation of the medical community, policy-makers, and the public. Third, given the difficulties expected in achieving such a broad-based consensus, it must adopt strategies designed to secure the support of the medical community and of policy-makers, and compliance by the public: i.e.

ensuring that the potential future rewards justify today's costs to policy-makers and real or perceived hardships to the public. Additionally, cancer prevention must focus on avoiding or reducing exposure to carcinogens, the cause of most cancers, rather than the current practice of *"Chemoprevention"* discussed earlier. There are several reasons for this. First, Chemoprevention consists of administering drugs expected to reduce the incidence or recurrence of cancer, especially in high-risk individuals, rather than to prevent cancer from developing in the population at large. Second, the mechanism of action of *"chemopreventive"* agents are ill defined and their long-term side effects can counteract their modest cancer-preventing benefits, as demonstrated in the Tamoxifen for Prevention of Breast Cancer study [3]. Moreover, because their long-term toxicity profiles are unpredictable, very large studies and decades of follow up would be required to establish their safety, efficacy, and risk-benefit ratio. Thus, applying the customary cancer drug development hit-and-miss approach to the search for cancer chemopreventive agents, as currently done, is likely to meet the same fate: decades of stagnation. In contrast, health policies designed to eliminate or reduce exposure to carcinogens at the individual and community levels constitute the first step in a three-prong cancer control approach that offers the best opportunity for progress in the War on Cancer. Moreover, implementing cancer prevention policies focused on the most lethal carcinogens first, as I propose, will ensure the most dramatic reductions in cancer incidence and mortality rates initially, a circumstance that will validate the well-grounded foundation of cancer prevention in the eyes of the public and of policy-makers, and ensure its longevity.

Some might argue, correctly, that we do not know how to prevent most cancers. However, to date a link has been established between cancer and the following etiologic factors (in descending order of their contribution to overall cancer incidence): Tobacco, obesity, viruses, alcohol, pollutants, radiation, genetic predisposition, and mutagenic drugs. Of these, tobacco, obesity, alcohol, and to a lesser extent exposure to ultra-violet radiation and carcinogenic viruses, are mainly life-style choices, often encouraged by beneficiary industries. Their control calls for behavioral changes by individuals supported primarily by appropriate motivational programs but also by compulsory legislation, when needed. In contrast, environmental cancer-promoting factors (mainly carcinogenic pollutants) are contributed mainly by the smokestack industry and by the entire community (mainly cars), and can only be curbed by enlightened policy-makers willing to assume leading and sometimes unpopular roles in the safeguard of public health. Finally, the control of cancers caused by inadvertent exposure to ionizing radiation, and to carcinogenic drugs, or resulting from genetic predisposition must address separate issues including environmental or workplace exposure, treatment risks, and human genetics, respectively. However, the purpose of this discussion is not to delineate a comprehensive national cancer prevention policy but to illustrate the enormous benefits of orienting such a policy according to its potential impact on cancer control. Thus, we elected to examine tobacco, the most lethal carcinogen, because curbing its use will have the greatest impact on cancer deaths in the US and worldwide. It also gives us the opportunity to examine the complicated and challenging behavioral issues on the part of individuals, corporations, and policy-makers that must be addressed and reconciled in order to bring about its control. We will also address exposure to carcinogenic viruses because although largely behavioral, as is tobacco use, their control is conceptually simpler and easier to implement in practice.

1.1   Tobacco

On October 12, 1492, Columbus noted in his journal *"The natives brought fruit, wooden spears, and certain dried leaves which gave off a distinct fragrance"*. A month later, Rodrigo de Jerez and Luis de Torres, two of Columbus' men, first observed smoking and reported that the Arawak Indians wrapped the dried pungent leaves *"in the manner of a musket formed of paper and after lighting one end, they drank the smoke through the other"*. Jerez took up smoking and is credited to have brought the habit back to Spain, but smoke spewing from his mouth and nose so frightened Spaniards, he was allegedly imprisoned by the Holy Inquisition. Legend has it that by the time he was released 7 years later, smoking was a Spanish craze [4]. Thus began the European tobacco saga that soon would find countless adherents around the world, given its growing social acceptance and alleged medicinal properties, its powerful addictive hold on users, and more recently the financial bonanza to cigarette manufacturers and to governments' tax revenues. However, with its 3,000-plus chemical components including at least 43 carcinogens, tobacco is the leading preventable cause of disability and deaths in the US and the world. As a major contributor to the four leading causes of premature death (heart disease, cancer, strokes, and chronic lung disease), cigarettes kill as many Americans as the next 10 causes combined, including: accidents, diabetes mellitus, influenza and pneumonia, Alzheimer's disease, kidney diseases, septicemia, suicide, chronic liver diseases, hypertension, and homicide [5,6]. In the US, illnesses attributable to smoking accounted for 430,000 premature deaths in 1990 [7] of which 189,700 were from cancer [8], representing approximately 20% and 30% of all premature non-cancer and cancer deaths, respectively [9]. Unless smoking patterns change drastically, worldwide mortality from tobacco is estimated to rise from 4 million deaths in 1998 to 10 million in 2030. Five hundred million persons alive today will eventually be killed by tobacco [10].

Given its carcinogenic components, a fact known by the tobacco industry as early as 1961[11], and because of smokers' long-term exposure, tobacco is the most lethal of human carcinogens. It is responsible for over 90% of lung cancers, the majority of cancers of the larynx, pharynx, oral cavity, and esophagus, and a substantial fraction of cancers of the pancreas, kidney, bladder, colorectum, and cervix [12,13]. Cigarette smoking was branded "*the major single cause of cancer mortality in the United States*" over 20 years ago, in the 1982 Surgeon General's report. However, despite national and local efforts to curb it, it retains its dominant position as the most hazardous cancer-promoting behavior, being responsible for nearly one in three cancer deaths [9]. Lung cancer alone, the cancer most directly and irrefutably linked to cigarette smoking, accounts for approximately 28% of cancer deaths in the United States [14]. Evidence that smoking cessation reduces disability and premature deaths is demonstrated by a 50% reduction in overall death rates within 10 years of cessation. This is contributed by a 50% reduction of coronary heart disease within 1 year, and a 50% decreased incidence of strokes and of cancers of the lung, the oral cavity, and the esophagus after 10 to 15 years of abstinence [15]. The net effect of 15 years of tobacco abstinence is a return to death rates enjoyed by persons who never smoked.

Despite obvious benefits, eliminating tobacco from our society will require a strong and sustained commitment by the medical community, policy makers, and the public who must overcome three levels of resistance. The first is the difficulty most smokers have in overcoming their addiction and their reluctance to exchange instant gratification for the prospects of a healthier and longer life. A typical smoker's excuse for defying a physician urging smoking cessation is, "*why live longer if I have to deprive myself of this daily pleasure?*" The second is the fierce resistance of cigarette manufacturers to abandon their cash cow, sustained by slick advertising to lure youngsters, their financial clout to influence policy-makers, and a cadre of prominent attorneys to defend their interests when challenged in the courts. The third is the willingness of politicians and policy-makers to sacrifice public health to the ambitions of a few including their own, at worst, or their unwillingness to adopt health policy based on good science rather than good politics, at best. Additionally, cigarette manufacturers have shown resourcefulness to counteract reductions in adult smoking in the US. They have concentrated their efforts mainly on three fronts: First, they have targeted American children through clever advertising. Second, they aggressively expanded abroad in some cases with the help of smugglers and money launderers, as alleged in lawsuits filed by European, Canadian, and Colombian state governments against Philip Morris and British American

Tobacco [16]. Third, they have shown willingness to resort to any means, including perjury before Congress, to resist adverse legislation. Hence, tobacco control must rely on sustained public educational campaigns enacted by enlightened policy-makers with the vigorous support and participation of the medical community. The Federal government must lead the way by abandoning its duplicitous policy of providing price support to tobacco growers (via the US Department of Agriculture) as it promotes anti-smoking activities (coordinated by the Centers for Disease Control and Prevention). Additionally, funding research in smoking-related illnesses (through the National Institutes of Health) on one hand, and unenthusiastic regulation of tobacco products (through the Federal Trade Commission, the Substance Abuse and Mental Health Services Administration, and the Food and Drug Administration) on the other, seems counterproductive.

To be effective, public campaigns should be broad-based to prevent initiation of tobacco use, promote cessation of use, and eliminate exposure to environmental tobacco smoke. Past experience indicates that such an approach yields substantial benefits [17]. For example, after rising from 54 cigarettes per capita in 1900 to 4,345 in 1963, the annual cigarette consumption in the US dropped to 2,261 per capita in 1998. Likewise, adult smokers decreased from 42.4% to 24.7% of the US population between 1964 and 1997, and persons who have never smoked increased from 44% to 55% between 1965 and 1997. These trends are responsible for the decline in lung cancer incidence and mortality in the US after 1991-1992. In large measure, these behavioral changes were encouraged by the first report of Surgeon General's Advisory Committee on Smoking and Health published in 1964 that concluded, "*cigarette smoking is causally related to lung cancer in men*". It was further reinforced by the 1982 Surgeon General's report that branded cigarette smoking as "*the major single cause of cancer mortality in the United States*". However, downward smoking trends stalled in the mid-1990s and today one in four Americans still smokes. More ominously, after decreasing through the 1980s to 30%, smoking among high-school seniors rose to 36.5% between 1991 and 1997 though it has slightly decreased since. During the same period, tobacco use has increased dramatically worldwide, leading the World Health Organization to establish the Tobacco-Free Initiative, and the World Health Assembly to approve unanimously, in May 2003 after nearly four years of negotiations, the Framework Convention on Tobacco Control at the global level. As of January 2004, 85 countries have signed the treaty but only 5 have ratified it. The United States has done neither [18]. Thus, the time has come to view tobacco and its industry for what they are: a lethal product with no redeeming value and anti-social merchants of death, respectively, and to act accordingly. If the US was able to mount a successful, concerted, and sustained nation-wide campaign to eradicate asbestos from the workplace, it should find the will and have the ability to unleash a similar assault on a product that causes one thousand times more disability and premature deaths than asbestos [21].

Powerful and enforceable tools to do so ultimately are in the hands of politicians and policy-makers. These include heavy taxation of tobacco products, banning all tobacco advertising, and outlawing contributions or donations in cash or other valuables by the tobacco industry or its representatives, directly or indirectly, to any person or entity, outside or inside government, especially themselves. At present, the national average excise tax per pack of cigarettes is $0.46 with South Carolina levying the lowest (7 cents), and New York and Washington the highest ($1.50 and $1.425, respectively) [19]. Studies on the impact of cigarette prices on teen smoking conducted at colleges and universities showed that a 10% price hike reduced adolescent smoking by 7%. Based on this ratio, it was calculated that increasing the cigarette tax by 43 cents per pack, as proposed by the defeated 1997 Hatch-Kennedy Senate bill, would have reduced smokers by 2.6 million and smoking-related premature deaths by 850,000 in the cohort of Americans age 18 or younger [19]. Likewise, the uneven restrictions imposed by state and local governments on smoking in public and work places [20] should be standardized and expanded to all states through Federal legislation.

In conclusion, tobacco kills as many Americans as the next 10 causes combined and accounts for nearly one third of all cancer deaths in the United States. Cumulative experience over three decades has shown that most patients with tobacco-induced cancers are diagnosed in inoperable stages for which no efficacious treatment exists. As a result, most patients die within one year of diagnosis, a figure that has changed little since 1973. On the other hand, there is unanimous consensus that anti-smoking campaigns, triggered by the 1964 US Surgeon General's report on the health risks of smoking, are responsible for reductions in cigarette consumption and the subsequent decline in lung cancer incidence and death rates in American males since 1992. Thus, despite the lukewarm nature and uneven application of tobacco-control measures enacted thus far, considerable progress is being made, providing proof of concept supporting this approach to cancer control. On balance, hope remains that spurred by the overwhelming scientific evidence of the health consequences of smoking and of the benefits of smoke-cessation, increasing numbers of individuals will respond appropriately. This includes smoking-cessation by smokers and the foresight, by the community at large, to elect policy-makers with a sense of duty and social responsibility, and the political courage to enact draconian legislative measures to curb the tobacco industry and eventually eliminate from society the most lethal of human carcinogens. If that comes to pass, upward of 500,000 premature deaths, half of them from cancer, will be prevented each year in the US, and countless more worldwide.

1.2   Cancer viruses

While tobacco control is a very complicated issue requiring behavioral changes by reluctant individuals and legislative action by hesitant policy makers to counteract the antisocial behavior of the tobacco industry, the control of carcinogenic viruses is in principle simpler, for it can be accomplished by immunization of populations at risk. Yet, its impact on cancer deaths worldwide would be enormous. Indeed, viruses proven carcinogenic to humans (HTLV-1 virus [22], Epstein-Barr virus [23], papillomavirus [24,] and certain adenoviruses [25,26]), are estimated to cause 15% of all cancers worldwide, including 80% of liver cancers and over 90% of cervical cancers [27]. These estimates will rise substantially should the suspected virus-link of several additional cancers be confirmed. The suspected links include Kaposi's sarcoma, brain, pharyngeal, and laryngeal malignancies, and several papillomaviruses, human herpes virus-8, polyoma virus, human endogenous retrovirus HERV-K, and simian virus 40.

Of all the human malignancies caused by carcinogenic viruses, liver cancer or hepatocellular carcinoma (HCC) is the most prevalent worldwide [28] and one of the most lethal, with survival rarely exceeding one year. HCC is the 5th most common cancer worldwide (560,000 cases annually), behind cancers of the lung (1,200,000), breast (1,050,000), colorectal (940,000), and stomach (870,000) [29]. However, it is the 3rd most fatal accounting for 8.8% of all cancer deaths, behind lung (17.8%) and stomach (10.4%) cancers. The major risk factors are exposure to hepatitis B and C viruses [30,31], which account for 80% of HCC worldwide [32], and to a lesser extent aflatoxin B_1, a fungus toxin associated with certain food staples, and vinyl chloride. Hemochromatosis, a rare genetic disorder, can also predispose to HCC. Despite the availability of a hepatitis B vaccine since 1981, there are currently 360 million hepatitis B carriers worldwide; most of who live in the underdeveloped world where the infection accounts for approximately 70% of HCC. Likewise, there are approximately 200 million individuals worldwide currently infected with the hepatitis C virus, of which there are 2.7 million chronic cases in the US and a similar number in Western Europe [33]. In industrialized countries, hepatitis C is responsible for approximately 70% of cases of chronic hepatitis, 60% of cases of HCC, and 30% of liver transplants [32,34], despite its lower prevalence and acquisition later in life than hepatitis B infection. Hepatitis B infection is endemic in Southeastern Asia especially in China, Taiwan, and Vietnam, where it affects 11.4% to 24.5% of the general population [32], whereas it is lowest in the industrialized world where prevalence is less than 5% of the population. In contrast, the highest incidence of hepatitis C occurs in Spain where 7.3% of the population is affected [33]. In underdeveloped countries, exposure to hepatitis B virus tends to occur at birth or in early childhood, while in industrialized countries the infection is usually contracted in adulthood. This early exposure, a 20% to 50% lifelong risk for developing HCC in hepatitis B-infected individuals, and an estimated 20 to 40 years interval between infection and the development of HCC explain the highest HCC incidence rates (90/100,000) in certain provinces of China where hepatitis B is endemic and acquired in childhood. In contrast, the lowest incidence of HCC (5/100,000) is recorded in Western Europe and the US [36] where hepatitis B is sporadic, begins in adulthood, and vaccination has been widely practiced.

Both hepatitis B and C viruses are transmitted percutaneously (IV drug use, infusion, transfusion, or transplant of infected materials, and occupational) or by permucosal routes (perinatal and sexual). In the US, the incidence of hepatitis B and C infections decreased sharply since the 1980s. This was due to behavioral changes on the part of homosexual men and IV drug users in response to the AIDS epidemics, to exclusion of tainted blood products that virtually eliminated that transmission route, and to the widespread use of hepatitis B vaccine promoted by the Occupational Safety and Health Administration. As a result, new cases of hepatitis C in the US have decreased over 90% since 1989: from approximately 140/100,000 to approximately 13/100,000 today [34,36]. At present, HCC ranks in 14th place among cancers in the US with approximately 18,920 new cases expected in 2004 [37] (Table I). However, given the lag time between viral infection and cancer development, decreasing infection rates will not translate into lowered HCC rates for another several decades, as has been the Japanese experience with hepatitis C. In that country, while the high incidence of hepatitis B and C after WWII was reduced dramatically in the 1980s and 1990s to levels matching the US and Europe, the incidence of HCC rose to a current 40/100,000, mostly in males over the age of 50, and is not expected to plateau for another 10 or 15 years [38]. Today, 80% of HCC cases in Japan are caused by hepatitis C infection, and 16% by hepatitis B. Similar rises in the incidence of HCC are expected to occur in industrialized countries, beginning with Spain and Italy where widespread hepatitis C virus infection already accounts for 70% and 48% of HCC cases, respectively. In the US, the incidence of hepatitis B peaked in 1985 with approximately 70 cases per 100,000 people, and hepatitis C infection peaked in 1989 with 140 cases per 100,000, forecasting a future rise in the incidence of HCC that is expected to peak between 2010 and 2020.

George Bernard Shaw's quote, *"As well consult a butcher on the value of vegetarianism as a doctor on the worth of vaccination"* suggests his unawareness of Pasteur's pivotal work on a rabies vaccine and his failure to foresee the future impact of vaccines on public health. In fact, the enthusiastic embrace of prophylactic vaccines by physicians, policy-makers, and the public has been unwavering. Massive immunization campaigns against childhood infections have sharply reduced the global incidence of diphtheria, whooping cough, tetanus, poliomyelitis, measles, mumps, rubella, and influenza. In the US, universal vaccination against these diseases has reduced their incidence by 95% to 100% since their peak a century ago [39]. More impressively, after 10 million people died of smallpox worldwide in 1966, the World Health Organization launched an eradication program of global scale that reduced the incidence of this disease to a single Somali case ten years later, leading the Organization to declare *"Smallpox is dead"* in May 1980 [40], three millennia after it killed the Egyptian Pharaoh Ramses V.

A recombinant form of hepatitis B vaccine is available worldwide, but none exists against the hepatitis C virus. The hepatitis B vaccine has proven safe and efficacious and one billion doses have been administered worldwide since 1982. It has shown to be 95% effective in preventing chronic infection in children and adults and, in certain areas where the prevalence of chronic infection was 8% to 15%, it has fallen to <1% of immunized children. In 1991 the WHO recommended that all countries add hepatitis B vaccine to their national immunization programs. However, ten years later 74 countries out of the 189 member states had not done so, most of them located in sub-Saharan Africa, the Indian subcontinent, and other poorest areas with the greatest need but devoid of the financial and infrastructure resources necessary to comply. To fill that void a coalition of private and public institutions, called the Global Alliance for Vaccines and Immunization, was founded in 1999 to fund childhood immunization programs against vaccine-preventable diseases, including hepatitis B, in the poorest 74 countries. Such vaccination programs will undoubtedly have a major impact on the incidence of HCC, especially in endemic areas, as suggested by the Taiwanese experience [41]. Ten years after implementing a nationwide neonate and toddler hepatitis B vaccination program, Taiwan recorded a 10-fold decline in the prevalence of chronic hepatitis B in children ages 6 to 14, along with a 43% decline in the incidence of HCC. It is therefore ironic that most current research in *"cancer vaccines"* focuses, not on prophylactic immunization against known carcinogenic viruses, but on vaccines designed to enhance the ability of the immune system to recognize alleged "*tumor antigens*" (MAGE, MART, CEA, HER-2, MUC-1, PSA and others), in attempts to mediate tumor rejection. Yet, after 20 years of attempts to coax the immune system to reject cancers using various forms of immunotherapy, only anecdotal successes have been reported. How are we to explain the enduring fascination of researchers with the concept of immunotherapy? The answer is multifaceted but includes three major factors. First is the intellectual attractiveness of extending the concept of immune rejection of *"non-self"* (bacteria, viruses, transplanted organs, etc) to cancer cells, even after the latter have been shown to be part of the *"self"* albeit harboring genetic alteration. Second is the intricacy of the immune system that challenges immunologists, molecular biologists, and geneticists interested in probing its multifaceted dimensions. Third is the anticipation of academic and financial rewards that are sure to accompany any genuine *"breakthrough"* in this domain, especially when compared to what is perceived as the uninspired endeavor of prophylactic anti-viral vaccine development.

In conclusion, known carcinogenic viruses account for approximately 15% of human cancers, an estimate that will rise substantially if several suspected but unproven virus-cancer links are confirmed. Experience to date indicates that most patients with virus-induced cancers are diagnosed in inoperable stages for which there is no efficacious treatment. As a result, most such patients seldom survive one year from diagnosis. On the other hand, prevention of HCC by hepatitis B virus vaccination offers the proof of concept that virus-induced cancers are preventable. Recent progress on papillomavirus vaccines [42-44] suggests that cervical cancer and other human malignancies induced by this group of viruses will soon be preventable. When this comes to pass, cervical cancer will become the first human malignancy to benefit from two of the three-prong approach to cancer control proposed in this book: prevention via prophylactic vaccination of women at risk and early-stage diagnosis via the reliable and cost-effective Papanicolaou's screening test followed by curative surgery. At that point, only unvaccinated women without access to health care, or through ignorance, poverty, cultural constraints, or self-neglect will be at risk of developing advanced-stage cervical cancer and face a grim prognosis. Given these results and the ease and cost-benefit ratio of immunization against carcinogenic viruses, it is incumbent upon researchers and their sponsors, particularly the NCI, to prioritize and fund the development and testing of prophylactic vaccines against all known carcinogenic viruses. Upward of 200,000 cancers could thus be prevented in the US each year and countless more worldwide.

2. CANCER SCREENING

Except for immunization against cancer-causing viruses, most cancer prevention programs entail long-term commitments to lifestyle and public policy changes of difficult implementation, reluctant participation by all parties involved, and deferred benefits. Thus, additional and complementary cancer control measures must include early detection of surgically resectable tumors and better therapies for patients with advanced cancer. At present, most cancers are diagnosed in relatively advanced stages or progress to advanced stages subsequently. Because the outcome of patients with advanced cancer is largely unaffected by current therapies, interest is growing among physicians, researchers, and the public regarding screening programs focused on early detection of cancer in asymptomatic individuals, when surgical cures and prolongation of survival are most likely. It must be stated at the onset that high-tech tools such as CT scans, MRIs, Flow cytometry, and molecular techniques are more useful for assessing the tissue of origin, stage, presence of metastases, and growth potential of a cancer, and to assess treatment responses or relapses, rather than for screening asymptomatic individuals. In fact, today's cancer-screening programs rely mostly on low-tech tests that are noninvasive, inexpensive, harmless, and simple to perform in the physician's office or at the local laboratory. However, being cancer non-specific these tests are unable to distinguish between malignant and benign lesions or between progressive and non-progressive tumors. Indeed, it is likely that much of the increased prostate and breast cancer incidence since the advent of PSA and mammography screening relates to the detection of lesions that while classified as cancers might never have progressed to clinical disease or cause morbidity. The uncertainty associated with the interpretation of screening test results was dramatized in a recent lay press article [45] addressing mammography, as follows *"You look for lumps and bumps, and you look for calcium. And, if you find it, you have to make a determination: is it acceptable, or is it a pattern that might be due to cancer?"* Not surprisingly, the inherent limitations and meager results achieved by current cancer screening tests have led to a controversy surrounding their usefulness. Nevertheless, the NCI and the American Cancer Society espouse cancer screening, and since 2000, the latter has issued updated guidelines for the early detection of breast, colorectal, prostate, and cervical cancers, as well as advice on risk avoidance and health maintenance measures [46]. I take the position that, notwithstanding the inadequacies of current screening tools, cancer screening is a conceptually viable means to control cancer. My position is based on the expectation that future cancer screening tools will emerge from mining the Human Genome database to understand the etiology and molecular biology of each cancer. From this viewpoint, to reject the cancer-screening concept outright amounts to throwing the baby with the bath water. Hence, the following section will review the current status of prostate and breast cancer screening based on three arguments. First, as the two malignancies with the highest incidence and second highest mortality rates in American men and women, prostate and breast cancer are ideal targets to impact national trends. Second, prostate and breast cancer screening has proven feasible at the community level and modestly beneficial. Third, these cancers also serve to illustrate the inadequacies of current cancer screening tools and the need for much progress in this area.

2.1   Prostate cancer

The American Cancer Society estimates that 230,110 cases of prostate cancer will be diagnosed in 2004 [37], the most common non-cutaneous malignancy in American men having [47,48] surpassed lung cancer by a ratio approaching or exceeding 2:1 since 1991. Yet, this places the US 22nd among world nations in prostate cancer incidence. Most prostate cancers progress slowly as shown by a 97% 5-year survival in the 1992-1998 period [48]. However, only 33% of patients with distant metastases reach that landmark, mainly due to the inefficacy of available treatment options (radical prostatectomy, external-beam radiation therapy, and brachytherapy). Inefficacious therapies and an extremely high incidence contribute to making prostate cancer the second leading cause of cancer-related death among American men in 1999 (31.5 /100,000 men), exceeded only by lung cancer (77.2 /100,000 men) [48]. This, and the observation that disease progression and patient survival are inversely proportional to primary tumor size [49], has focused attention on the need for early stage diagnosis through screening. At present, there are three methods for prostate cancer screening: digital rectal examination (DRE), prostate-specific antigen (PSA), and transrectal ultrasound (TRUS) which is mostly relegated to guiding prostate biopsies in individuals with an abnormal DRE or PSA.

Although DRE has been used for many years, systematic evaluation of its usefulness for prostate cancer screening has not been undertaken and several studies of different design and goals have been less than encouraging. For example, in a 1984 study of 811 elderly men, 38 of 43 with abnormal DRE underwent prostate biopsy. Of these, 11 or 29% had cancer, but 56% of them were locally or distally invasive [49,50]. Other studies that raised doubts about the DRE procedure for early-stage detection include the following: only 20% of prostate cancers were localized to the gland when diagnosed following annual DREs [51]; 25% of individuals with metastatic disease at the time of diagnosis had had a normal DRE [52]; and a comparable number of individuals had undergone DRE during the previous ten years among 150 men who ultimately died of prostate cancer and 299 controls without disease [53]. Thus, while DRE is noninvasive, inexpensive, and simple to perform in the physician's office, it is not a dependable screening tool to detect early-stage disease.

In contrast, the PSA test has the advantages of being operator-independent, objective, and more sensitive. Its widespread use in the US since the late 1980s led to an explosion in incidence rates of prostate cancer, mostly indolent types. Age-adjusted incidence rates rose evenly from 1973 to 1986 but nearly doubled between 1987 and 1992, peaking at 235.9 /100,000 men in 1992 [48]. This rise resulted from the increased use of transurethral prostatectomies [47], but mostly due to the widespread use of the PSA test [54,55]. On the other hand, mortality rates rose only modestly and steadily between 1974 and 1991 without paralleling the explosive rise in incidence rate after 1987. This is mainly because a large portion of tumors detected by PSA are early-stage or non-progressive cancers, or are lesions that are not cancers in the biologic sense, all associated with good prognosis. After a sharp decline in incidence rates during the 1992-1995 period and a gradual but modest drop in mortality rates between 1993 and 1998, both rates have remained unchanged [48]. These statistics imply a positive impact of PSA screening on early-stage diagnosis and mortality rates, and several prospective studies have confirmed the relationship [56-58].

Perhaps the most compelling evidence derives from a PSA mass-screening program in the Federal State of Tyrol, Austria. Out of 65,123 men aged 45 to 75, 32.3% were tested the first year and over two thirds were tested at least once during the first five years of the program. Registry records show a shift towards early-stage disease and an increased proportion of organ-confined disease, a trend previously reported in the U.S. by the SEER program, also in conjunction with PSA use. Mortality rates from prostate cancer dropped from 1993 onward at a faster rate in Tyrol than in the rest of Austria where no screening took place [56], though the increased utilization of diagnostic biopsies during the pre-PSA era had already begun the shift toward early-stage diagnosis and increased survival. Similarly, declines in the number of cases with advance disease and in mortality rates were also reported from Olmsted County in Minnesota and from a Department of Defense prospective population study. Together with the Tyrol experience, these studies support the view that screening for prostate cancer saves lives. Finally, combining PSA and DRE appears to increase cancer detection as shown by the largest PSA/DRE screening study [57]. In this study, 22,014 out of 116,073 men screened were found to have an abnormal PSA, DRE, or both. Prostate cancer detection was 4.5%, when DRE and PSA were used in combination, compared to 2.5% for DRE alone [58]. Based on this evidence, the American Cancer Society developed sound guidelines on prostate cancer screening: A PSA test and DRE should be performed annually on men age 50 with a life expectancy of at least 10 years. Men at high risk (men of African descent or with first-degree relative diagnosed at a young age) should be tested from age 45. Men with multiple first-degree relatives diagnosed with prostate cancer at an early age should commence testing at age 40 (if the initial PSA is less than 1.0 ng/dl, no further testing is necessary until age 45). PSA values between 1.0 ng/dl and 2.5 ng/dl should trigger annual testing, and a PSA above 2.5 ng/dl should be considered grounds for a biopsy. While a 2.5 ng/dl PSA cut-off value (as compared to the *"normal"* cut-off value of 4 ng/dl) increases detection of prostate-confined cancers, it also increases the number of false-positives (cancer-free biopsy), and procedure-associated morbidity. Thus, the guidelines also emphasize the importance of a having a fully informed patient who participates in the decision-making process: a bewildering prospect for many anxious patients facing cancer. Yet, mass screening for prostate cancer is being resisted in some quarters based on three arguments. First, as a cancer-nonspecific test, PSA cannot distinguish between benign and malignant lesions. Second, it cannot establish the progressive or indolent nature of a malignancy. Third, it cannot predict whether an individual will survive long enough to be at risk for disease morbidity and mortality. While these arguments are valid they should encourage a search for better screening tests rather than be used to dismiss the cancer-screening concept as a viable cancer-control measure.

In conclusion, prostate cancer is the most common non-cutaneous malignancy in the US with almost a quarter of a million new cases expected in 2004. While most prostate cancers progress slowly, treatment for advanced disease is inefficacious and patients rarely survive more than 5 years from diagnosis. As a result, prostate cancer is the second cause of cancer mortality in American men, accounting for approximately 10% of cancer deaths. On the other hand, the massive, multi-year PSA screening program conducted in the Austrian province of Tyrol and two studies in the US increased detection of early-stage cancers and reduced mortality rates in PSA-screened men. These data provide the proof of concept supporting the use of PSA in population screening programs aimed at reducing prostate cancer mortality. However, because PSA is not a cancer-specific screening test it is associated with a substantial number of inconclusive results that require a biopsy for clarification and cause additional morbidity, and leads to treatment of lesions that might never have progressed to clinical disease. Thus, cancer-specific screening tests must be developed to differentiate benign from malignant lesions, and to establish whether an early-stage tumor is indolent or is likely to progress to clinical disease within the life span of a particular patient, thus justifying therapeutic intervention with potential morbidity

2.2   Breast cancer

Breast cancer is the most common non-cutaneous cancer among American women, though it is even more common in 15 European countries. In the US, 217,440 new cases are expected in 2004, with fewer than 1,500 occurring in men [5] (Table I). The reported incidence of breast cancer increased at an annual rate of approximately 1% between 1940 and 1980, but 4% between 1980 and 1987, probably because of prior life-style changes and the widespread use of mammography screening [59]. Since then, the rise in incidence has stabilized at less than 0.5% annually. A woman's chance of developing breast cancer increases with age from 1 out of 257 between age 30 and 40, to 1 in 25 between age 70 and 80, which translates to a 1 chance in 8 risk of breast cancer over her lifetime. Breast cancer was the leading cause of cancer-related death in American women through 1998, when it was surpassed by the steady and rapid rise in lung cancer mortality. The American Cancer Society forecast that 39,800 women will die of breast cancer in 2003 [5]. Mortality rates remained fairly constant (approximately 32/100,000 women) between 1973 and 1990, and decreased subsequently at an annual rate of 1%. While this is multifactorial, a major contributor is the detection of asymptomatic, early-stage disease associated with favorable prognosis [59]. In contrast, prior to the widespread use of screening, breast cancer was frequently diagnosed in advanced stages, when a woman sought medical counsel for symptoms or a self-discovered mass [60]. At present, there are three widely used breast cancer-screening tools: breast self-examination (BSE), clinical breast examination (CBE), and mammography.

Monthly BSE has been advocated despite an absence of convincing evidence of its effectiveness. For example, in one large study of retired textile workers in Shanghai, China, 267,000 women age 30 to 65 were randomized to receive or not instruction in BSE [61]. A high level of compliance and proficiency was achieved in the BSE group through reinforcement sessions and multiple reminders. After a 5-year follow up period, more benign breast lesions were detected in the BSE group (1,457) than in controls (623), suggesting a higher index of suspicion by trained women. However, approximately equal numbers of breast cancers were detected in the two groups (331 in the BSE group and 322 in the control group). Likewise, tumor size and stage were similar in the BSE and control groups, as were the cumulative mortality rates (30.9/100,000 and 32.7/100,000, respectively). Other studies have confirmed that BSE does not reduce the risk of advanced breast cancer [62,63] or breast cancer mortality [63]. Like BSE, a breast examination performed by a physician (CBE) is routinely practiced in the US and elsewhere despite conclusive evidence of its usefulness as a breast cancer-screening tool. For example, a very large study

[64] that analyzed 752,081 CBEs in community settings demonstrated the superiority of mammography. In that study, the cancer-detection rate was 7.4 per 1,000 cases with an abnormal CBE but a normal mammogram, 42/1,000 for the combination normal CBE/ abnormal mammograms, and 170/1,000 when both were abnormal. This study demonstrates that almost 1 in 5 cancers detected by mammography escaped CBE detection.

Mammography is the most studied and, having yielded better results than BSE or CBE, the most frequently used in the clinical setting. However, it too has serious limitations: its sensitivity and specificity depend on factors such as lesion size and conspicuity, breast tissue density, patient age and hormonal status, image quality, and the interpretative skill of the radiologist. In order to minimize the effect of some of these factors and to ensure quality and safety, in 1992 Congress enacted the Mammography Quality Standards Act that empowers the FDA to exercise regulatory control over any facility offering mammography. This has led to improved techniques, to more efficient equipment with lower radiation exposure, and to better trained personnel. Yet, a retrospective study of 183,134 screening mammograms revealed that while sensitivity (detection of cancer when cancer is present) in women age 65 and older reached 81% to 94%, it remained in the mid-50% in women under 40 [65]. Another study found that 150 breast cancers not detected during a 5-year screening period but diagnosed within 24 months of the last mammogram, afflicted women under 50 and were more aggressive [66]. However, rather than questioning the validity of mammography, these findings indicate that initially undetected aggressive cancers can develop quickly. They also suggest that the interval between screening tests should be different for indolent and progressive cancers, an imponderable that can only be established in retrospect. Finally, a critical factor affecting the accuracy of mammograms remains radiologists' level of expertise. For example, two studies revealed that several radiologists interpreting the same films rightly recommended additional work-up in 75% or greater of women whose breast cancer were diagnosed shortly after their mammograms [67,68]. However, they also tended to over-interpret mammograms of women who did not develop cancer [69], especially if prompted by a suggestive clinical history [70].

The above limitations notwithstanding, clinical trials have shown that cancer survival is better in mammography-screened than unscreened women. However, while this survival advantage is believed related to detection of cancer in early stages, other factors might play a role. These include a healthier life-style of women who adhere to a screening program; the added survival (lead-time bias) associated with early diagnosis; and the favorable impact of more cases of indolent cancers diagnosed with than without mammography. The likelihood of diagnosing breast cancer is highest with the first screening, ranging from 9 to 26 cancers per 1,000 mammograms, compared to 1 to 3/1,000 with subsequent screening [71]. The aggressive nature of cancers arising between screening examinations [66] underscores the importance of re-screening. Yet, the optimal interval between screening procedures is not known and might not matter much given the aggressive and rapidly progressive nature of such cancers. Added to these imponderables are the issues of false negative and false positive results, and of radiation exposure. Mammograms detect cancer in only 0.1% to 0.5% of women at the time of screening [71] and miss 1 in 5 cancers, a fact not generally known by health care professionals or the public that often leads to legal action and to large awards to plaintiffs. Alternatively, false-positive mammograms often lead to additional procedures to delineate the nature of an abnormality, including repeat mammograms with magnification of the suspicious area, ultrasound, fine needle aspiration, and core biopsy. These additional procedures cause a heavy toll in terms of anxiety, discomfort, morbidity, and cost, especially because most abnormal mammograms prove benign on further investigation. For example, the cumulative risk of false-positive mammograms was ascertained retrospectively in 2,400 women age 40 to 69 enrolled in a health maintenance organization for 10 years [72]. During that period, a total of 9,762 screening mammograms and 10,905 screening CBE were performed. The estimated cumulative risk of a false positive result was 49.1% after 10 mammograms and 22.3% after 10 CBE. False positive tests led to 870 outpatient appointments, 539 diagnostic mammograms, 186 ultrasound examinations, 188 biopsies, and 1 hospitalization. It was estimated that for every 100 dollars spent for screening, an additional 33 dollars was spent to evaluate the false positive results. In another study [73], evaluation of abnormal mammograms in 23,172 elderly women revealed that for every 1,000 women, 85 had follow-up testing including 23 biopsies. Thirteen percent of women had repeat mammograms more than once, and 11% of women undergoing breast biopsies had more than one such procedure. Interestingly, concern that further testing of false-positive mammograms might dissuade women from future examinations was put to rest by several studies that have shown just the contrary [74]. It seems that such an experience may increase a woman's determination to undergo regular screening. Finally, concern has also been raised about radiation exposure as a risk factor for future breast cancer, especially in young women. However, for women age 40 or older the benefits of annual mammograms outweigh the potential risk of radiation exposure, especially given the low dose delivered by modern equipment.

Doubts have also been expressed regarding the extrapolation of results of randomized trials in a research setting to the community practice setting. This view was supported mainly by a highly controversial meta-analysis of eight randomized clinical trials conducted on nearly 500,000 women in 4 countries (US, Canada, Sweden, and Denmark) between 1960 and 1980 comparing breast cancer mortality in women offered or not screening. The authors found flaws in 5 of the 7 studies and concluded that the evidence did not support screening mammography [75]. However, after an exhaustive review of the same data by the U.S. Preventive Services Task Force (USPSTF), the US Department of Health and Human Services Secretary Tommy Thompson released, on February 21, 2002, an updated recommendation advising screening mammography every 1-2 years for women ages 40 and over. A week later, appearing before a combined US Senate Committee Andrew von Eschenbach, M.D., Director, NCI stated, *"We have reviewed the evidence and the USPSTF recommendation, and we conclude that the weight of the evidence shows that mammography saves lives through early detection and treatment at an earlier stage"* [76]. Demonstration that mammographic screening reduces breast cancer mortality in women participating in clinical trials has been extended to the community setting. In one study, evaluation of mammography screening in two Swedish counties showed a 63% decline in mortality from breast cancer diagnosed in screened women ages 40 to 69 during the screening period (1988-1996) when compared to breast cancer mortality during an equivalent time span preceding screening (1968-1977) [77]. A second, more recent, and more extensive analysis of the effect of organized mammographic screening programs on breast cancer morality was undertaken in 7 Swedish counties, where approximately one third of the Swedish population lives [78]. This report demonstrated that mammography-screened women experienced a 44% reduction in breast cancer mortality when compared to mortality rates during the pre-screening period and a 39% mortality reduction when compared to non-participating women during the screening period. Based on its interpretation of the cumulative evidence, the American Cancer Society has recently issued a new update [79] to its initial 1992 guidelines for the early detection of breast cancer. Bucking this evidence, it recommends that women begin monthly BSE at age 20, an annual CBE between 20 and 39, and beginning at age 40, an annual CBE quickly followed by a mammogram so that a mass detected by CBE is brought to the attention of the radiologist. In contrast, the US Preventive Services Task Force reaffirmed the value of mammography leading HHS Secretary Tommy Thompson to announce, *"The federal government makes a clear recommendation to women on mammography: If you are 40 or older, get screened for breast cancer with mammography every one or two years"*.

In conclusion, in the US breast cancer will afflict 1 in 8 women during their lifetime and, despite decades of attempts to improve its treatment outcome, it is the second cause of cancer mortality in American women today, accounting for approximately 15% of cancer deaths. This is because breast cancer, like most malignancies, is often diagnosed in advanced, inoperable stages for which treatment is less than optimal. As a result, most such patients seldom survive more than a few years from diagnosis. On the other hand, the best evidence to date has shown that mammography with or without BSE or CBE is a modestly effective tool for the early detection of breast cancer in surgically curable stages, especially in older women. This and reductions in mortality rates for mammography-screened women provide the proof of concept supporting the use of mammography in population screening programs aimed at reducing breast cancer mortality. However, like PSA, mammography is a cancer-nonspecific screening tool that is associated with a substantial number of inconclusive results that require a biopsy for clarification and cause additional morbidity, and leads to treatment of lesions that might never have progressed to clinical disease. Thus, medical researchers should focus on developing more sensitive screening tools of greater specificity capable of distinguishing between benign and malignant lesions and of identifying aggressive forms of cancer from indolent types that might never cause morbidity. Such tools would considerably reduce the discomfort, anxiety, morbidity, and cost associated with additional procedures required today for making that distinction. In the meantime and until prevention and efficacious treatments for advanced prostate and breast cancers become available, early detection with all its faults, offers improved chances for survival to the 1 in 8 American women and 1 in 6 American men, and millions more around the world, who will face breast and prostate cancer over their lifetime.

3.   WHEN PREVENTION AND SCREENING FAIL: A NEW CANCER TREATMENT PARADIGM

Even the most comprehensive cancer prevention campaigns cannot be expected to eliminate cancer, nor can the best screening programs detect all cancers is early, curable stages. Additionally, the development and implementation of effective nation- and worldwide prevention and screening policies will take time. Thus, for the foreseeable future, many cancer patients will continue to exhibit advanced-stage disease when first diagnosed or progressive disease and, under the cell-kill paradigm, inevitably die of it. However, we now have the knowledge and the opportunity to improve this somber outlook for future patients. It requires repudiating the cell-killing paradigm that has dominated the War on Cancer, and anchoring future treatment strategies on targeting the molecular and genetic defects that govern the emergence, growth, and dissemination of cancer cells. The new strategies need not lead to the abrupt abandonment of all present forms of chemotherapy, but to their progressive replacement by specifically targeted agents that prevent, reverse, or control the molecular or genetics defects that underlie each cancer type, as they become available. It also requires a massive redirection of funds and the training of a new breed of clinical researchers to abandon the cell-kill paradigm and its corollaries and to focus their attention on targeting the abnormal signaling pathways underlying cancer development and progression. Only then will we bridge the ever-widening gap between the science of cancer and its clinical management.

The first and most formidable hurdle will be to engineer a repudiation of the entrenched mind-set by clinical cancer researchers illustrated by the following announcement by NCI: "*The ongoing challenge in cancer drug design remains the same: to develop drugs that are effective at killing tumor cells without unnecessary damaging healthy tissue*" [80]. Examples of future cancer therapy cited in that document include immunotherapy that "*seeks to boost, direct, or restore the body's own cancer-fighting mechanisms*", and cancer vaccines that "*stimulate the immune system to recognize antigens on the cancer cells, eliciting an immune response against those cells*". Both approaches imply a continued adherence to the misguided notion that cancer cells are fundamentally different from their normal counterparts, and the possibility of their selective recognition and elimination by a "supercharged" immune system. It is noteworthy that while immunotherapy as conceived today is mediated by the organism's own defense mechanisms to maintain the integrity of the *self*, its goal remains firmly anchored in the cell-killing concept of cancer therapy; the aim being to kill cancer cells. However, awakened by the remarkable success of Imatinib mesylate in controlling rather than killing its targeted malignant cells, on February 16, 2000, NCI belatedly invited "*exploratory/developmental grant applications to exploit molecular targets for drug discovery*". It also announced, "*Rather than depending on in vitro and in vivo screens for antiproliferative activity, investigators can now focus on new molecular targets and pathways essential for the development and maintenance of the cancer phenotype. As a result, the NCI is reorganizing its drug development programs from early drug discovery phases to the conduct of clinical trials in order to bring forward new types of agents based on strong rationales*" [81]. However, not yet prepared to break with the past, on August 22, 2002 the NCI announced a drug discovery program based on analytical software designed to correlate patterns of NCI-60 growth inhibition by more than 80,000 chemical compounds with microarray-based NCI-60 gene expression [82]. While this approach is likely to accelerate discovery of cancer-inhibitory or broadly cytotoxic drugs it will not necessarily identify carcinogenic targets crucial to the molecularly targeted control of cancer. In contrast to the NCI's still pregenome approach, the future of cancer drug development rests on post-genome pharmacogenomics, which essentially inverts the process. It identifies the genetic defects underlying cancer, delineates their role in the carcinogenic pathway, and then seeks drugs suitable to block or control the abnormal function of the cancer-causing genes. Although more rational than the pre-genomic hit-and-miss approach to drug development, today's nascent pharmacogenomics is an uncertain and equally unpredictable undertaking. Indeed, it requires deciphering normal and abnormal cell signaling. Yet, our rapidly increasing knowledge of these intricate events has revealed that what were once thought to be simple one-way pathways are in fact multidirectional, redundant, and recurrent. Nevertheless, two lines of arguments suggest their future necessity and feasibility. First, while worldwide research funding by the drug industry has more than doubled since 1991, drug discovery has dwindled. For example, only 21 "*new molecular entities*" (entirely new rather than modified drugs) were approved by the FDA in 2003 vs 53 in 1996. Second, Imatinib mesylate a "*designer*" drug that targets the bcr/abl protein product provides the proof of concept of how this strategy can succeed.

3.1   The bcr/abl fusion gene: a prototypic molecular target

The discovery of oncogenes, in addition to providing valuable insights into the nature and regulation of cancer cells, led to the development of tools for diagnosing and monitoring cancer at the molecular level. Moreover, oncogenes and their protein products represent potential targets for highly specific molecular therapies of cancer. One of the best-known oncogenes is the so-called "*Philadelphia*" chromosome. First described by Nowell and Hungerford in 1960, it was quickly identified as the chromosomal abnormality that characterizes CML [83]. Later shown to represent a translocation between the long arms of chromosomes 9 and 22, detection of the Philadelphia chromosome became a hallmark to confirm a clinical diagnosis of CML in the practice setting. In this disease the c-abl gene, normally located at 9q34 (band 34 of the long arm of chromosome 9), is translocated to 22q11 (band 11 of the long arm of chromosome 22) where it becomes fused with the bcr gene. Depending on the bcr breakpoint, several chimeric (recombined) mRNA molecules can result that translate into chimeric fusion proteins 210kd (p210) or 185kd (p185) in length. p210 is expressed by approximately 95% of adult CML patients and half of the approximately 25% of adult cases of acute lymphoblastic leukemia (ALL) bearing the bcr/abl fusion gene. In contrast, a smaller fusion protein (p185 or p190) is expressed by 80% of the 5% of cases of childhood ALL and the other half of the adult ALL bearing the bcr/abl fusion gene. The chimeric protein encoded in the bcr/abl fusion gene exhibits tyrosine kinase activity that, through the activation of various intracellular signaling pathways, alters the adhesive and survival properties of host cells and confers onto them a proliferative advantage. bcr/abl has been clearly documented as the sole leukemogenic abnormality using mice transgenic for p185, and irradiated mice repopulated with hematopoietic stem cells expressing the p210 [84,85].

The bcr/abl chimeric gene exhibits many characteristics of an ideal therapeutic target: it is present in 95% of cases of adult CML, it causes the disease, and the cell-transforming function of its encoded protein is mediated by an activated tyrosine kinase. This constellation of attributes made it clear that inhibitors of tyrosine kinase could be extremely effective and highly specific therapeutic agents for the treatment of CML. The search for such compounds began in the late 1980s and eventually led to the synthesis of STI571 or imatinib mesylate, now commercialized in the US under the name Gleevec®. After preclinical studies demonstrated the in vitro and in vivo activity against bcr/abl-expressing cells, STI571 entered clinical studies in 1998. In a dose-escalation Phase I study, STI571 at 300 mg or greater induced a complete hematologic remission in 98% of 54 patients with CML that was maintained in 96% after a median follow up of 310 days, with only mild side effects [86]. More importantly, the estimated rates of complete cytogenetic response were 76.2% [87], raising the possibility of an eventual eradication of the malignant CML clone. Cytogenetic remissions of this magnitude have never been recorded using other therapies. The study was expanded to include CML patients in myeloid (n=38) and in lymphoid (n=20) blast crisis. Responses were observed in 55% and 70% with blast clearance in 21% and 55%, respectively. However, the duration of response was less than 4 months in nearly all patients with lymphoid blast crises and less than12 months in 82% of patients with myeloid blast crises. In phase II clinical trials, over 1,000 patients with chronic, accelerated, or blastic phase CML were accrued at 27 centers in 6 countries [88]. This large study confirmed both high remission rates with little toxicity and an inverse correlation between disease phase and the rates of hematologic remissions, cytogenetic responses, and duration of response. The best results occurred in the chronic phase and the worst in the acute phase of the disease, especially of the lymphoid type. Despite its clear advantages, STI571 is not universally efficacious for the treatment of CML. In some patients, STI571 fails to inhibit the tyrosine kinase activity. This usually results from increased drug efflux, bcr/abl amplification, additional kinase mutations, and other factors [89,90] that render the bcr/abl insensitive to the inhibitory effect of STI571. In other cases, kinase inhibition fails to induce a response or relapses occur in spite of continuous inhibition of the kinase. This can result from additional molecular mutations that drive the malignant clone, aside from the bcr/abl [91,92].

Although CML was an ideal disease target for testing the anti-cancer efficacy of STI571, this agent was originally developed against the platelet-derived growth factor (PDGF-R) and was later shown to inhibit the c-kit tyrosine kinase as well. This observation generated considerable interest because numerous cancers express these therapeutic targets. PDGF-R is expressed in glioblastoma, chronic myelomonocytic leukemia, non-small cell lung and breast cancer, seminoma, and myelofibrosis and other fibrotic conditions. C-kit is expressed in gastrointestinal stromal tumors (GIST), small-cell lung cancer, acute myelocytic leukemia, neuroblastoma, melanona, mastocytosis, and other cancers [93]. However, the role of PDGF-R and c-kit in the pathogenesis of these diseases is unclear, expect in GIST, mastocytosis, seminoma, and possibly some cases of acute myeloid leukemia where they appear to be causative [94]. Of these, GIST, a highly refractory malignancy expressing activated c-kit showed a 60% response rate in phase I clinical trials, whereas those with wildtype or inactivated c-kit proved less responsive [95].

From these cumulative clinical observations, three major lessons can be drawn to guide future molecularly targeted therapy. First, cancer therapy should be directed to specific molecular cancer-causing targets rather than to specific types of cancer: that is, treatment should be based on genotype rather than on phenotype. Second, the effectiveness of molecularly targeted agents should be judged by their biological effect on targets rather than by the usual tumor-size reduction criteria ingrained in the cell-kill paradigm. Third, molecularly targeted cancer therapy will be most successful when a single genetic abnormality drives the malignant clone. In cases where more than one mutation contributes to clonal survival and progression, clonal control will require preventing genomic instability or curbing each abnormality identified as causative. Preventing or controlling unstable genomes and hence the incremental genetic abnormalities resulting from dysfunctional cell cycle gate-keepers is but one form of molecularly targeted therapy. The attractiveness and potential reward of this approach is highlighted by the fact that unstable genomes are common denominators to cancer progression regardless of the initial cancer-causing genetic defect. Their stabilization would prevent or control cancer progression and dissemination, hence enabling the sustained efficacy of molecular therapy targeting the primary carcinogenic defect. Yet, the complexity of such a task underscores the relative simplicity of cancer prevention and screening in comparison.

In conclusion, CML is the first human malignancy demonstrably caused by a genetic abnormality: the bcr/abl chimeric gene. It is also the first to be controlled by a molecularly targeted drug (Imatinib mesylate) specifically developed to block the gene-encoded protein that confers leukemic cells their survival and proliferative advantage, without cell-kill. This provides the proof of concept supporting the feasibility of using molecularly targeted drugs designed to reverse or control the genetic defects responsible for the development, growth, and dissemination of cancer. With Imatinib mesylate the new era of pharmacogenomics is launched, and with it a new paradigm for the treatment of cancer. At present no other cancer causing genetic abnormality has been identified, but a vigorous search already underway in hundreds of research laboratories worldwide, will in time be fruitful. Hence, the shift from cytotoxic to gene-targeted therapies will and must be incremental. Yet, it promises to be a difficult and massive undertaking that will call for a radical transformation of the pharmaceutical industry, cancer research, and patient care, as discussed in the next chapter.

3.2 The genome and proteome as bases for anti-cancer drugs

At the outset, it must be acknowledge that we stand at the threshold of knowledge in cancer genomics. Yet, once the difficulties of deciphering the human genome database are overcome, translational applications in the clinical setting promise to revolutionize drug development and the future treatment of human ailments, including cancer [96,97]. However, to do so will require comparing normal and cancer genomes on a comprehensive and massive scale, facilitated by the human genome sequence completed in April 2003, with delineation of the intron-exon boundaries for all human genes, concluded in 2004. This knowledge is necessary to dissect the genetic bases of the biologic hallmarks of cancer (self-sufficient production of proliferative signals, insensitivity to growth inhibitory and apoptotic signals, limitless replicative potential, promotion of angiogenesis, invasion, and metastases), to understand the functional interactions of these genes in the development and progression of cancer, and to exploit that knowledge for drug development and patient care. The initially estimated 100,000 human genes has been lowered to 30-40,000, raising concerns that the anticipated 6,000-10,000 drug-targeted genes [98] might also have to be revised, though this view has been challenged [99]. This is because identification of a cancer gene does not necessarily translate into a pharmaceutically tractable or "*druggable*" target, as is the case of tumor suppressor gene p53, also known as the guardian of the human genome. As the most commonly lost or mutated cancer gene responsible for tumor resistance to cytotoxic drugs, p53 is one of the best-characterized and understood cancer genes and therefore an ideal targetable gene. However, reversing a loss-of-function mutation has proven highly challenging. Indeed, attempts to re-introduce wild-type p53 into tumor tissues [100], or to inoculate the tumor with a cytolytic virus that replicates selectively in p53-deficient cancer cells in order to kill these cells [101] have met with limited success. Similarly, disruption of cancer promoting and cancer sustaining protein-protein interactions such as Myc-Max and Ras-Raf dimers has proven difficult because the potency, pharmacokinetics, or safety profiles of candidate peptides were not suitable for human use. Yet, the proof-of-concept demonstrating the feasibility of genotype-specific, oncogene-based, targeted cancer treatment arose from the clinical success of a monoclonal antibody specific against the Her2 gene product that is over-expressed in 30% of breast cancer patients [102]. Approved in 1998 by the FDA for the treatment of Her2-positive breast cancer under the brand name Herceptin ®, this agent induces 60% to 70% responses when combined to paclitaxel [103] or doxorubicin in this subgroup of patients, though the latter combination is more cardiotoxic [104]. Clinical experience with Imatinib mesylate in bcr/abl-expressing tumors and with Herceptin in Her2-positive breast cancer amply confirms the validity of the strategy of basing cancer drug development on cancer genetics. These successes have encouraged a large array of preclinical and clinical studies using anti-estrogen receptors, protein kinase inhibitors, Ras farnesylation, matrix metalloproteinases, integrins, antibodies, antisense oligonucleotides, viruses against potential genomic targets [105,106], and gene therapy [107]. Targeted areas of intense interest include apoptosis, signal transduction pathways, tumor growth factors, angiogenesis, and cell cycle control.

In conclusion, fully decoding the human genome and understanding how mutated genes functionally interact in the development, progression, and dissemination of cancer will enable the translation of that knowledge into the identification and validation of new cancer drug targets for patient care. Additionally, it will generate genotypic profiles underlying diagnosis, prognosis, treatment response, and susceptibility to toxicity. Finally, it will facilitate developing complementary or alternative means to strategically circumvent intractable targets or clinically unsuitable candidate molecules in the drug development process, and to overcome cancer genome instability, a hallmark of progressive cancers. While the task is daunting and will prove arduous, complicated, and costly, it also provides the first rational and evidence-driven foundation upon which to build an approach to successfully treat advanced cancer.

Chapter 13

SHIFTING FROM THE CELL-KILL PARADIGM TO PHARMACOGENOMICS

Delineation of cancer genomes on a comprehensive scale and large-scale translational applications will require the concerted efforts of the research community as well as substantial public support. The initial phases of this elaborate and massive undertaking has already benefited from the efforts and vast human and financial resources of the public and private sectors. However, given their divergence in goals and motives, the molecularly targeted drug development phase, an endeavor dominated by private industry, is likely to favor profit-driven tracks. In such a scenario, targeted drugs likely to be pursued vigorously will be those with the highest financial return on investment. Thus, the focus, at least initially, will be on drugs for cancers with high incidence rates and those relatively inexpensive to bring to market. Cancers with genetic defects not easily *druggable* or with low incidence rates among the population will be shunned or disfavored. Another area of concern is whether the medical community and the public are prepared to abandon the notion of cancer as an "invader" to be eradicated at all cost and to embrace the view that it results from genetically dysfunctional cells that can be brought back to a normal life cycle ending in apoptosis. Likewise, assessment of the efficacy of gene-targeted drugs and of treatment response must shift from the cancer cell-kill paradigm to biological surrogates of tumor response. As suggested by experience with Imatinib mesylate, molecularly targeted cancer drugs are likely to have a low toxicity when compared to current cytotoxic cancer drugs, which commonly lead to life-threatening myelosuppression and immunosuppression. This and their modulating rather than cytotoxic mechanism of action should help focus clinicians' attention on patient outcome rather than tumor outcome, as is currently the case under the cell-kill paradigm. However, a new cancer management strategy that emphasizes the functional control rather than the destruction of cancer cells is such a radical departure from the current cancer-eradication dogma that its implementation will require re-educating clinical researchers, community physicians, patients, and the public at large.

1.   A BLUEPRINT FOR FUTURE CLINICAL CANCER RESEARCH

It is clear that cancer control will undergo a progressive transition, from a purely cytotoxic era based on the pre-genomic concept of cell-kill, to prevention, to early-stage diagnosis, and to post-genomic, gene-targeted drugs designed to reverse or control the molecular abnormalities that render a normal cell malignant. That is, future cancer agents will modulate genetic targets that are causally involved in the development, progression, and dissemination of cancer. Completion of the human genome sequence, followed by the identification and characterization of cancer genomes will accelerate target discovery and its corollary, pharmacogenomics. This transition will accelerate the ongoing industrialization of molecular biology, transform molecular diagnostics at the industrial and clinical levels, metamorphose the pharmaceutical sector, and ultimately revolutionize cancer care. Recognition that genetic mutations are associated with a predisposition to certain diseases has contributed to an explosion of increasingly sophisticated technologies intended to identify genetic polymorphism accurately, swiftly, and cost-effectively. As refinements in genetic and molecular techniques develop, cancer gene expression profiling will uncover biological relationships with clinical relevance. The most promising new technologies are designed to decipher and exploit genome sequences. They include high throughput screening, nanotechnology, robotic science, combinatorial chemistry, proteomics, and gene expression microarrays. These techniques, combined with informatics and database mining, will accelerate identification of targetable molecular defects and drug development. Numerous biotechnology companies have emerged to capitalize on a large and potentially profitable market for specific, accurate, yet easily applied and cost-effective products for research or clinical use. Undoubtedly, the day will come when genetic testing kits will diagnose a variety of diseases or detect, in a few minutes for a few dollars and with great accuracy, gene expression profiles [108,109]. These tools will enable predicting disease predisposition, response to therapy, susceptibility to side effects, and other biological variables embedded in a person's genes.

Yet, initial resistance to change is to be expected given the prevailing attitude that "*Many but not all drug companies, mindful of profits, prefer the easy way out and concentrate on analogues, while most clinicians opt for trials of combinations of known agents, being aware that they are worth a publication or two"* [110]. However, the well-grounded foundation of the concept of molecularly targeted medicine and its potential benefits in cancer management, as highlighted by the therapeutic success of Imatinib mesylate, will convert individual and corporate skeptics alike. Community Oncologists will enthusiastically embrace target-specific drugs with greater efficacy and lower toxicity, especially given public support and demand for novel agents touted in the media as *"miracle"* drugs. The pharmaceutical industry will be compelled to rethink its tendency to reach as large populations as possible, the *"blockbuster"* drug development model, and adopt strategies to develop drugs that target specific molecular pathways designed to address the needs of small populations most likely to benefit. While such strategies will likely increase drug development costs that are difficult to amortize given their smaller customer base, the expected increased specificity and efficacy of gene-targeted drugs and the commonality of genotype targets across dissimilar disease phenotypes present unique business opportunities. For example, while Imatinib mesylate was developed against a chimeric gene responsible for CML it has also shown efficacy against phenotypically dissimilar tumors that involve similar genetic abnormalities. Will these drugs be affordable? Certainly, the high complexity of the modern drug development process, both at the technical and regulatory levels, increases costs. However, demands for expanding government health care funding in rich countries, pressures on the pharmaceutical industry for greater accountability, and rising living standards in the developing world should markedly increase the demand for and affordability of future cancer drugs in direct proportion to their efficacy.

The efficacy of Imatinib mesylate against phenotypically dissimilar malignancies suggests that the transition will be accompanied by an evolution of the current diagnostic approach from a histologic- to a molecular-based model. Such a re-classification of malignancies, according to their underlying genotype rather than their external phenotype, is fundamental to the generation of a cancer genome database as a foundation for developing and validating gene-targeted drugs. The therapeutic relevance of uncovering molecular diversity within phenotypic homogeneity and vice versa has already been validated in some cancers using chromosomal analysis. For example, patients with acute promyelocytic leukemia expressing the translocation t(15:17) respond to all-trans retinoic acid and to arsenic trioxide, whereas the other phenotypic subtypes of acute myeloid leukemia do not [111]. Likewise, patients with chronic lymphocytic leukemia harboring an unmutated IgVH gene exhibit a more progressive disease with a worse prognosis than those with a mutated IgVH gene locus despite otherwise similar clinical and laboratory profiles [109]. This method of supervised genetic clustering using a known point of departure (the chromosome, gene, or sequence of interest), will likely give way in the future to unsupervised clustering methods. In the latter case, automated robotic analysis of large-scale gene expression experiments is undertaken to identify and classify sequence groups directly from the raw database [110].

The transition from a phenotype- to a genotype-based classification of cancer will demand a new level of interactions among biologists, computer scientists, biostatisticians, and clinicians. This will be necessary in order to generate, store, analyze, and interpret the massive amounts of genetic data that will emerge from the new high throughput techniques required for identifying and validating potential drug targets, target-modulating drugs, and biologic markers of therapeutic endpoints, and for designing appropriate clinical trials. From these general considerations, broad guidelines for future clinical cancer research begin to emerge. First, there will be a migration from cytotoxic drugs that target phenotypically similar cancers to cytostatic drugs that target genotypically related cancers regardless of their anatomic origin or histologic features. Second, by reversing or controlling the genetic defects that underline malignant cells, future cancer drugs will curtail their growth or survival advantage and lead to an orderly, genetically controlled implosive apoptosis without sequels. Third, new models must be developed to identify and validate molecular targets, target-specific drugs, novel diagnostic and prognostic assay systems, and new clinical trial designs. Each will require surrogate endpoints of efficacy designed to assess and validate the biologic effects of post-genomic drugs in vitro and their efficacy in the clinical setting.

Identification of a molecular target is but the beginning of a long discovery process that ranges from gene profiling to pharmacogenomics to clinical trials. The latter pose particular challenges to clinical investigators. This is in part because the traditional concepts of maximum tolerated dose and tumor response endpoints that have guided Phase I and Phase II trials of cytotoxic drugs are not suitable to assess the efficacy of targeted drugs given their specificity and genotype-modulating mechanisms of action. Thus, new ways to assess efficacy will be needed. This is largely due to the fact that through inhibiting the growth or survival advantage of cancer cells, gene-targeted drugs will attempt to restore these cells' pre-cancerous growth potential, lifespan, and apoptotic pathway without cell-kill. Under these circumstances the degree of tumor size reduction will relate more to the growth rate and apoptotic deregulation of cancer cells than to the extent of their functional restoration. For example, agents that curtail cell division or accelerate cell death, such as tyrosine kinase inhibitors [86-88], farnesyl transferase inhibitors [112], antibodies [102,103], and certain gene therapies [107], can induce appreciable tumor shrinkage in cancers with rapid growth rates or markedly decreased apoptosis. However, new biological endpoints as surrogates of tumor and clinical responses must be developed to judge biological response and restoration of cell function. Ideally, biological endpoints should derive from and be linked to the drug effect on the molecular target. For example, in the case of Imatinib mesylate, inhibition of tyrosine kinase can be judged by falling white blood cell counts and by reductions in the proportion of malignant cells in blood and bone marrow. However, a constellation of favorable circumstances makes CML an ideal rather than a typical candidate for targeted drug studies. These include clinical (i.e. white blood cell count) and biological end-points (i.e. chromosome analysis) that are technically easy to monitor in readily accessible blood and bone marrow specimens with little risk or discomfort to patients. Easy access to tissue samples has fostered rapid progress in cancer genetics and gene profiling of hematologic malignancies, which will be the primary beneficiary of translational research, at least initially. This is not the case, however, for solid tumors given an absence of identifiable causative genetic defects and their generally deeply seated anatomic location that precludes repeated tissue sampling.

In attempts to bypass such limitations, surrogate tissues and surrogate markers are being actively sought, especially for deep-seated tumors. An ideal surrogate tissue should be accessible easily and repetitively, in abundant quantities, and with minimal discomfort and risk to patients. Such an approach is illustrated in a phase I trial conducted in 20 patients with extensive solid tumors to assess SCH66336, a farnesyl transferase inhibitor that inhibits H-ras and K-ras-4B farnesylation in vitro [113]. Buccal mucosa cells were chosen as surrogate cells to examine processing of farnesylation-dependent prelamin A as a potential marker of in vivo activity of the SCH66336. While none of the buccal smears contained prelamin A before treatment, this marker was detected in increasing percentages of buccal mucosa samples in a direct proportion to the dose of SCH66336 administered, thus validating the concept of surrogate tissue for that drug model. However, to be reliable a surrogate marker must also quantitatively mimic the anti-cancer effect of a drug. This was brought to light in a phase I trial of O^6-bensylguanine in-patients with locally advanced or metastatic cancer [114]. O^6-bensylguanine inhibits the enzyme O^6-alkylguanine-DNA alkyl transferase (AGT) responsible for resistance to alkyl nitrosoureas. AGT levels in surrogate blood cells were nearly depleted 18 hours after infusion of 10 mg/M^2 of O^6-bensylguanine, whereas a comparable effect on tumor tissues obtained via computed tomography-guided biopsies, required 120 mg/M^2. This study highlights but one of the potential difficulties of finding reliable tissue or marker surrogates. In addition to the search for marker and tissue surrogates, non-invasive approaches are being investigated especially positron emission tomography that measures metabolic cell activity as means to discriminate between normal and neoplastic tissues and to monitor treatment response. However, the potential and role of these instruments remains to be determined.

Finally, because current phase II clinical trials are not valid to assess post-genomic drug efficacy, novel designs have been proposed [115-118] to identify and validate molecular targets and targeting drugs, to translate that information to the clinical setting, and to assess results of clinical trials. While many challenges remain, the anticipated benefits of future pharmacogenomic drugs amply justify pressing forward, particularly given decades of near stagnation under the pre-genomic cell-kill paradigm that dominated clinical cancer research and patient management.

2.   A BLUEPRINT FOR FUTURE PATIENT MANAGEMENT: PROPORTIONAL AND COMPASSIONATE

The transition from cytotoxic to molecularly targeted cytostatic drugs will be accompanied by a shift in cancer treatment from a tumor-centered to a patient-oriented approach. This combined strategy is based on three sets of facts. First, long-term experience indicates that cancer eradication using non-specific cytotoxic drugs is a flawed concept with a mostly unachievable goal. Second, the expectation that the future of cancer therapy lies in controlling the aberrant molecular genetic pathways responsible for the development, growth, and dissemination of cancer, rather than trying to killing the cells that harbor them. Third, the absence of direct correlation between tumor size reduction and survival, which suggests that the efficacy of genomic drugs will be judged by their effect on survival and other patient-related end-points. A patient-oriented rather than tumor-centered approach to cancer management has the added advantage of focusing physicians' attention on patients' multi-dimensional needs and to respond accordingly. These needs are not addressed currently, as highlighted by the National Cancer Policy Board report entitled *"Improving Palliative Care for Cancer: 2001"* [119]. This report was launched in response to, among others, a Robert Wood Johnson Foundation study that criticized the medical community for not providing adequate care to cancer patients approaching the end of life. The report examined the scientific, policy, and social barriers that keep those in need from getting adequate palliative care, and recommended ten public- and private-sector initiatives to develop effective palliative interventions and ensure access to palliative care for all eligible cancer patients. The co-editor of the report stated, in her June 19, 2001 public briefing, *"In the pursuit of a cure, the nation has almost ignored the need to reduce the suffering by physical and emotional symptoms of cancer and side effects of cancer treatment...it is important to emphasize that while we work to cure the many different kinds of cancer, nothing would have a greater impact on the daily lives of cancer patients and their families than good symptom control and supportive therapies"*. Indeed, numerous surveys of terminally ill patients have indicated that medical treatment is often inconsistent with patients' preferences [120]. Patients usually emphasize receiving adequate pain and symptom relief, avoiding prolongation of dying, achieving a sense of control, and strengthening relationships with loved ones. In a recent survey [121], 40% of 1,185 seriously ill Medicare patients expressed a preference for treatments designed to prolong life and in 86% of them their wish was honored. However, only 41% of those who preferred comfort measures thought their preferences were honored. Of the 40% who received unwelcome aggressive therapy, 55% were dead within one year suggesting once again the futility of misguided attempts to prolong life, as symptom control was being neglected. The magnitude of unnecessary and preventable suffering by terminal cancer patients can be surmised from the following statistics: 50% to 84% of the more than 500,000 Americans who die of cancer each year complain of at least one symptom [122], especially during the active phase of treatment [123].

The notion that the individual's welfare is the overriding principle guiding all medical treatments has its roots in the Hippocratic Oath pledged by physicians upon graduation. It states in part, *"I will follow that system of regimen which, according to my ability and judgment, I consider for the benefit of my patients, and abstain from whatever is deleterious and mischievous"*. Today, Oncologists' *"ability and judgment"* benefit from a factual knowledge and a clear understanding of the risks and benefits of each chemotherapy drug and of each drug combination, enabling them to assign curative therapies to patients afflicted by curable cancers and appropriately adapted palliative care to the rest. However, the curative model of cancer management is so ingrained in the US that in practice most patients with advanced cancers, even those with types that over decades of clinical trials have demonstrated refractoriness to cytotoxic drugs, receive chemotherapy. Moreover, chemotherapy frequently escalates from *"first-line"* to equally toxic but usually less efficacious *"second-line"* and finally *"salvage"* therapy, a euphemism used for last resort regimens that rarely salvage anyone. Generally, only when the available drug armamentarium has been exhausted, intolerance precludes further treatment, or death is near are patients referred to a hospice program for end-of-life palliative care.

This widespread, self-reinforcing attitude has been tacitly endorsed by a report of the Outcomes Working Group of the American Society of Clinical Oncology that recommended *"In the case of metastatic cancer, treatment can be recommended even without an improvement in survival, if it improves quality of life"*. Even as it acknowledged that, *"patient outcomes should receive higher priority than cancer outcomes"*, it added, *"multiple outcomes should be considered because no single outcome adequately describes the results of cancer treatment"*. This implicit carte blanche extended to Oncologists, the self-appointed arbiters of what constitutes a treatment response often with the acquiescence or resignation of hopeful or desperate patients, has fostered the perverse use of toxic drugs in attempts to enhance quality of life. Undoubtedly, as stated in the WHO definition of palliative care, *"Radiotherapy, chemotherapy and surgery have a place in palliative care, provided that the symptomatic benefits of treatment clearly outweigh the disadvantages"* [124]. For example, radiation therapy is used appropriately as an adjunct to control bone pain from multiple myeloma or metastatic bone disease, or to relieve circulatory or respiratory complications of invasive lung cancer. Likewise, chemotherapy can be successful in controlling constitutional symptoms in an otherwise refractory patient with non-Hodgkin's lymphoma, and surgical excision of an intestinal tumor is often advisable to forestall future bowel obstruction in a patient with an otherwise unresponsive cancer. However, extending the definition of palliative care to cytotoxic chemotherapy given to patients without the prospect of survival prolongation or symptom relief, as frequently done, is to rationalize treating patients whose outlook is unlikely to change. This constitutes a distortion of the concept of palliation and leads to additional burden but few redeeming benefits.

As defined by the World Health Organization, palliative care is *"the active total care of patients whose disease is not responsive to curative treatment. Control of pain, of other symptoms, and of psychological, social and spiritual problems is paramount. The goal of palliative care is achievement of the best possible quality of life for patients and their families. Many aspects of palliative care are also applicable earlier in the course of the illness, in conjunction with anticancer treatment"* [124]. Thus, palliative care should not be construed as synonymous with non-curative treatment or restricted to end-of-life Hospice care, but be viewed as an integral part of a patient-focused management strategy to begin at the time of diagnosis. Palliative care is concerned not with death but with the quality of life until death, particularly in terminally ill patients whose needs are not only physical but acquire psychological, familial, social, and spiritual dimensions. However, given Oncologists' emphasis on the relentless pursuit of tumor responses rather than patient outcomes and the toxic nature of cancer drugs, especially used in maximum tolerated doses to increase efficacy, treatment complications are common while meaningful benefits are few. This can be avoided by upholding the principle of proportionality that ensures that potential risks are commensurate with and justified by potential benefits. For example, the risk of life-threatening infection or bleeding associated with aggressive treatment of acute myelocytic leukemia in a young adult with a favorable cytogenetics profile and no co-morbidities is amply justified. This is because 72% of such patients survive 5 years if treated compared to a 4 to 6 months if left untreated [125]. However, an individual with one of many malignancies customarily refractory to cytotoxic chemotherapy and with no reasonable expectations of a prolonged survival would be ill advised to embark in a potentially life-threatening treatment.

Thus, an ideal palliative care plan should ensure, first and foremost, omission of futile or otherwise inappropriate therapies that augment patients' pain and suffering without offsetting benefits, and second, a commitment to adequate palliative care of disease symptoms and unavoidable treatment-related side effects. While there are gray zones between potentially beneficial and futile therapies, adherence to the principle of proportionality provides a useful practical guide in the treatment decision process. Such a point of departure does not restrict cancer treatment to the types of cancer that are amenable to a cure or to a prolongation of survival. Instead, it serves as a beacon for assessing the suitability of the type, intensity, and duration of treatment, especially for patients who have failed to respond to first-line, standard of care management. Such an approach sanctions treatment of all eligible patients with first-line, standard of care therapies, thus benefiting the occasional patient whose unusual response to therapy lay outside the "*means*" for generally unresponsive types of cancers. It also acquiesces to an occasional patient's request to continue a failed treatment while a personal or family landmark is reached. However, by definition "*outlying*" treatment responses are not representative of the majority for whom the treatment is ineffective. Such cases should not be used as an indication of the efficacy of a particular treatment modality, or as a basis to treat additional patients with similar clinical profiles. Likewise, chemotherapy undertaken solely to maintain hope, console relatives, or postpone the day when both patient and physician must contemplate and address the prospects of imminent death would be eliminated. However, perhaps the most useful feature of this approach is to raise barriers to today's treatment escalations for unresponsive cancers, from first-line to equally or more toxic second-line and then to salvage regimens, eventually exhausting all applicable treatments or the patients' physiological or emotional tolerance. This widespread practice is indefensible when applied to patients with indolent and asymptomatic disorders, such as chronic lymphocytic leukemia or low-grade lymphomas, whose overall survival, often comparable to the general population's, remains unaffected despite transient tumor size reductions or short tumor-free periods [126].

In conclusion, given the somber reality that a cure or a meaningful prolongation of survival are not currently attainable outcomes for most patients afflicted by advanced-stage cancers, treatment should be guided by the principle of proportionality. This principle emphasizes non-maleficence and ensures that expected treatment benefits, gauged by patient outcomes rather than by tumor outcomes, always outweigh potential risks. Adoption of this principle as the guidepost for safeguarding and promoting patient welfare would be a major advance in the delivery of suitable, competent, and compassionate cancer care. This is especially relevant to cytotoxic chemotherapy but is also applicable during the transition to cytostatic therapies. It will remain relevant as long as we continue to rely on relatively inefficacious but toxic cancer drugs. However, the dual principles of proportionality and non-maleficence will remain suitable and desirable standards for cancer therapies of the future. Indeed, while future anti-cancer drugs will likely be less toxic than today's, they are unlikely to be completely devoid of side effects regardless of mechanism of action.

CONCLUSIONS

The *War on Cancer* was given impetus by the *National Cancer Act of 1971*, which tapped the vast resources of the Federal government to confront the growing cancer challenge. As a result, all cancer initiatives funded by Federal dollars have been channeled through the NCI; itself remade by the National Cancer Act. While proponents who anticipated the conquest of cancer by the nation's bicentennial were overly optimistic and patently unrealistic, this book reviews the achievements and failures of the *War on Cancer* in an objective and dispassionate manner, based on factual data published in mainstream scientific journals and other reliable sources. Over four hundred pertinent, easily retrievable, and verifiable references are cited in support of the author's core argument that the *War on Cancer* has been lost, and of his proposed three-part approach to cancer control as an alternative to the failed cell-kill dogma that dominated clinical research and patient care for decades.

First, we must acknowledge that the *National Cancer Act of 1971* has had a profound and multifaceted positive impact on basic cancer research. However, translational application of our growing understanding of the nature of cancer to patient care has lagged far behind. Indeed, while our knowledge in molecular biology and genetics of cancer has grown exponentially in the last 20 years, patient care has improved only marginally despite the National Cancer Act. This is mainly due to neglecting prevention, undervaluing screening, and to our over reliance on inefficacious non-specific cancer drugs stumbled upon by serendipity or developed by a process of trial-and-error favored by the NCI, the main drug development funding source until recently. For example, molecular genetics is now poised to uncover the genetic defects underlying the emergence, growth, and dissemination of each of the more than 200 human cancers. In contrast, the

181

17 drugs identified by the World Health Organization as *"essential"* to manage cancer were developed between 1953 and 1983. Less than a handful of drugs developed since then is having a meaningful impact on cancer care. As a result, in 2003 fewer than 24,000 Americans with mostly advanced hematologic or embryonal cancers, representing approximately 2% of all cancers, were cured of their disease by chemotherapy used alone or in combination with surgery or radiation therapy. In contrast, over 550,000 Americans died of cancer that same year despite receiving a variety of cytotoxic drugs, often to the very end. Of these, over 150,000 or 28% of all cancer deaths died of tobacco-induced lung cancer, the most lethal though preventable malignancy in the US and worldwide, after an average survival of 7 to 8 months; a figure virtually unchanged since 1973.

Thus, how are we to interpret reports of declining cancer incidence and death rates in the US after 1992 and of increased survival over decades? Is progress finally being made in cancer treatment? Unfortunately, the fall in incidence and mortality rates after 1992 did not extend beyond 1995 and 2000, respectively. Moreover, in 1997 fewer patients died of cancers with decreasing mortality rates (39% of total cancer deaths) rather than with increasing mortality rates (51% of total cancer deaths), and 86% of the decline was due to reduced death rates in only 5 cancers. Additionally, factors other than treatment have contributed to lower mortality rates after 1992, and to increased survival over several decades. While the latter is due mostly to improvements in overall health care over time, the former resulted from public education campaigns that foster prevention via reduction in environmental and behavioral risk exposure, and early stage diagnosis via screening programs. Overall, fifty years of cytotoxic chemotherapy contributed minimally to the modest improvements in mortality rates or survival. This is because the faulty cell-kill paradigm, that views cancer as a *"new growth"* distinct from the host that must be eradicated at any cost, has misguided drug development and patient care for decades. From a treatment standpoint, surgery can satisfy this overriding principle because of its ability to remove early-stage cancer visually discernible from neighboring normal tissues, but current cancer drugs cannot given their non-specific mechanism of action unrelated to the cancerous process. This, in large measure, explains why innumerable attempts to enhance the efficacy of cytotoxic drugs, mainly via drug combinations and dose escalation with or without bone marrow transplantation, have failed to substantially increase cure rates or prolong survival for most cancer patients. That being the case, why does this failed system endure? The answer is multifaceted but can be summarized in one sentence. The information pipeline, generated by clinical researchers and supported by their sponsors and publishers, fosters standards of care that are reinforced by financial incentives and the extraordinary capacity of physicians for self-delusion, and by unrealistic expectations of consumers nurtured by the media.

Thus, the time has come to abandon the cell-kill paradigm and to anchor cancer control on an incremental, three-tier approach that incorporates prevention, early diagnosis, and when these fail, on controlling the aberrant genetic defects that lead to the development, growth, and dissemination of cancer. Is this approach likely to succeed where the cell-kill paradigm failed? It could be argued that, while found flawed in retrospect, past cancer control strategies seemed sound when first advocated, suggesting that the new paradigm I propose might also lead us astray. However, in contrast to hypothesis-driven past strategies the present proposal is solidly anchored on proof of concept for each of its components. Prevention has been validated by the success of anti-smoking campaigns in reducing the incidence of lung cancer in American males and by hepatitis B immunization programs in reducing the incidence of liver cancer in Taiwan. Screening programs to uncover cervical, prostate, and breast cancer in surgically curable early stages are saving lives, though screening tools at our disposable today are insensitive, non-specific, and confined to only a few cancers. Finally, the feasibility of controlling aberrant genetic defects underlying cancer rather than killing the affected cells has been amply demonstrated by the efficacy of Imatinib mesylate, the first specific, molecularly targeted anti-cancer agent of the post-genomic era. However, treatment of advanced cancer will remain at a disadvantage relative to prevention and early-stage diagnosis given the sheer size and greater genetic deregulation of such tumors. Ultimately, the success of the proposed measures will require a strategic shift from reliance on the conceptually faulty and implementally failed cell-kill notion of cancer treatment to a post-genomic cancer control paradigm. The new paradigm calls upon medical researchers to design means to identify and prevent cancer-causing agents, to develop simple, specific, and cost-effective screening tools for the early detection of all cancers, and to exploit the vast genomic database towards translational therapies for patients with advanced or progressive malignancies. It also calls upon policy makers to enact enlightened public policies towards cancer prevention and screening programs of national scope and achievable goals, and for the NCI to play a pivotal role in steering funding towards prevention, screening, and translational research. At the community level, it urges practitioners to focus on patient- rather than tumor-outcomes, to ensure that potential treatment risks are justified by the probability and magnitude of expected benefits, and to provide maximum pain relief and comfort to terminal patients.

REFERENCES

PART I & II

1. Ries LAG, Kosary CL, Hankey BF, et al. Editors. SEER Cancer Statistic Review, 1973-199. Bethesda, MD: National Cancer Institute, 1999.
2. National Heart, Lung, and Blood Institute. Fact Book Fiscal Year 2002. www.nhlbi.nih.gov/about/02factbk.pdf.
3. McGeary M, Burstein M. Sources of cancer research funding in the United States. Prepared for National Cancer Policy Board, Institute of Medicine. June, 1999.
4. Jemal A, Tiwari RC, Murray T, et al. Cancer Facts & Figures 2004. CA Cancer J Clin 2004; 54:8-29. http://www.cancer.org/docroot/STT/stt_0.asp
5. Ries LAG, Eisner MP, Kosary CL, et al. SEER Cancer Statistics Review, 1975-2000, Natl Cancer Inst. Bethesda, MD, http://seer.cancer.gov/csr/1975_2000/.pdf
6. Resident population estimates of the United States by Age and Sex: April 1, 1990 to July 1, 1999, with short-term projection to November 1, 2000 U.S. Bureau of the Census, Washington, D.C. 20233, http://www.census.gov/population/estimates/nation/intfile2-1.txt
7. Percy CL, Miller BA, Ries LAG. Effect of changes in cancer classification and the accuracy of death certificates on trends in cancer mortality. *Ann NY Acad Sci* 609:87-97,1990.
8. Swan J, Wingo P, Clive R, et al. Cancer surveillance in the United States: Can we have a national system? *Cancer* 83:1282-1291,1998.
9. Surveillance, Epidemiology, and End Results. About SEER http://seer.cancer.gov/about/
10. SEER Program (www.cancer.gov) SERR*Stat Dataase: Incidence - SEER 9 Regs Public-Use, Nov 2002 Sub (1973-2000), National Cancer Institute, DCCPS, Surveillance Research Program, Cancer Statistics Branch, released April 2003, based on the November 2002 submission.

11. Landis SH, Murray T, Bolden S, et al. Cancer Statistics, 1999. CA Cancer J Clin 49:8-31,1999.
12. Thun MJ, Wingo PA. Cancer Epidemiology in Holland-Frei, eds. Cancer Medicine ^{e.}5, 2000. http://www.cancer.gov/downloads/PUB/DOCS/SECTION4/23pdf
13. Estimated US Cancer Prevalence. http://cancercontrol.cancer.gov/ocs/prevalence/prevalence.html#survivor
14. Devesa FS, Silverman DT, Young JL, et al. Cancer incidence and mortality trends among whites in the United States, 1947-84. *J Nat Cancer Inst* 79:701-770,1987.
15. Nomura A. Stomach cancer. *In*: Cancer epidemiology and prevention, 2nd ed. Schottenfeld D, Fraumeni JF, editor. New York; Oxford University Press; 1996 p707-724.
16. Gann PH. Interpreting recent trends in prostate cancer incidence and mortality. *Epidemiology* 8:117-119,1997.
17. Welch HG, Schwartz LM, and Woloshin S. Are increasing 5-year survival rates evidence of success against cancer? *J Am Med Assoc* 283:2975-2978,2000.
18. Black WC and Welch HG. Advances in diagnostic imaging and overestimation of disease prevalence and the benefits of therapy. *N Engl J Med* 328:1237-1243,1993.
19. 2001 Cancer Progress Report, http://progressreport.cancer.gov/
20. Arias E, Anderson RN, Hsiang-Ching K, et al. Deaths: Final data for 2001. National vital statistics reports: vol. 52 no 3. Hyattsville, MD: National Center for Health Statistics. 2003. http://www.cdc.gov/nchs/data/nvsr/nvsr52/nvsr52_03.html.
21. Centers for Disease Control and Prevention. National Center for Health Statistics, http://ea.grolier.com/ea-online/wsja/text/ch08/tables/lv/27.htm
22. National population projections III Population pyramids 1990-2100, http://www.census.gov/population/www.projections/natchart.html
23. Jemal A, Thomas A, Murray T, et al. Cancer Statistics, 2002 CA Cancer Clin 52:23-47,2002. http://www.cancer.org/downloads/STT/CancerFacts&Figures2002TM.pdf
24. US Cancer Statistics Working Group. United States Cancer Statistics: 2000 Incidence.Atlanta (GA): department of Health and Human Services, Center for Disease Control and Prevention and National Cancer Institute; 2003.
25. SEER Cancer statistics Review 1973-1997 Table I-3, Summary of changes in cancer incidence and mortality, 1950-1997 and 5-year relative survival rates, 1950-1996.
26. SEER Cancer statistics Review 1973-1998, Table I-2 (49-year trends in US cancer mortality rates).
27. Kardinal CG, Yabro JW. A conceptual history of cancer. Sem Oncol 6:396-408, 1979.
28. Hippocrates, Aphorism #38 Book 6
29. Celsus AC. De Medicina, book 5, Chapter 8.
30. Aetius of Amida, Book 14, chapter 4. Edited by Janus Cornarius, Venice 1534

31. Galen C. On tumors beyond nature, Chapter 13.
32. Wolf J. The Science of cancerous diseases from earliest times to the present. Science History Publications USA, 1989 pg12.
33. Andreae Vesalii Bruxellensis, scholae medicorum Patavinae professoris, De humani corporis fabrica libri septem. Basilae: Joannis Oporini (printer), Mense Junio, 1543.
34. Ambroise Paré, (a brief biography) http://ambroise.pare.free.fr/
35. Paré A. In Hamby WB. The Case Reports and Autopsy Records of Ambroise Paré. Springfield, IL: C.C. Thomas; 1960 [As cited in Shimkin MB, Contrary to Nature: Cancer, p. 57 (q.v.)].
36. Cited by Wolff Jacob, in The Science of cancerous disease from earliest times to the present. Science History Publications, 1989, p42
37. Descartes R. Discours de la méthode pour bien conduire sa raison et chercher la vérité dans les sciences, 4e partie, 2e Méditation.
38. Aselli G, De lactibus sive Lacteis venis, 1627
39. Bett WR: Historical aspects of cancer, in Raven RR (ed) Cancer, vol I. Butterworth, London 1957, pp 1-5.
40. Petit J-L. Oeuvres completes, Limopes 1837, pg 438 (cited in Wolf J. The Science of cancerous diseases from earliest times to the present. Science History Publications USA 1989, pg 50.
41. Petit J-L. Essai sur le cancer des mammelles, cited by Darmon P, in Les céllules folles, Plon, Paris 1993.
42. Peyrhile B. Dissertatio academica de cancro, Lyon, 1773 (cited in Wolf J. The Science of cancerous diseases from earliest times to the present. Science History Publications USA 1989, pp 54-55).
43. Ramazzini B. De Moribus Artificum Diatriba. 1713. [Translation by Wright WC reprinted in Birmingham, AL: Classics of Medicine Library; 1983
44. Griffiths, M. Nuns, virgins, and spinsters: Rigoni-Stern and cervical cancer revisited. British Journal of Obstetrics and Gynecology. 98:797-802,1991.
45. Hill J. Cautions against the immoderate use of snuff and the effects it must produce when this way taken into the body.London: R. Baldwin & J. Jackson
46. Bayle GL et Cayole. Cancer, in Dictionnaire des sciences médicales, Pankouke, Paris, 1812, vol III, p 671.
47. Broca PP. Mémoire sur l'anatomie pathologique du cancer. Bulletin de la Société anatomique de Paris, 1850, 25: 45 et seq.
48. Virchow R. Die Cellular pathologie, 1858.
49. Velpeau AALM. Traité des maladies du sein, Paris 1853.
50. Remak R, described in Muler's Archiv, 1852, p 57, as quote in Wolf J. The Science of cancerous diseases from earliest times to the present. Science History Publications USA, 1989, p182.
51. Bard L. Anatomie générale des tumeurs, Lyon 1895.
52. Boveri T, Zur Frage der Entstehung maligner tumorem, 1914.
53. Holmes OW. Currents and countercurrents in medical science, with other addresses and essays (Boston: Ticknor and Fields, 1861), p. 39. cited in Parascandola J. From germs to Genes: Trends in drug therapy, 1852-2002. Pharm Hist 44(1):3-11,2002

54. Peller, S. Cancer research since 1900. An evaluation. Philosophical Library, New York, 1979.
55. Fibiger JAG, The Nobel Prize in Physiology or Medicine 1926, http://www.nobel.se/medicine/laureates/1926/index.html
56. Asghar RJ, Parsonnet J. Helicobacter pylori and risk for gastric adenocarcinoma. Semin Gastrointest Dis 12(3):203-8,2001
57. Seto M. Genetic and epigenetic factors involved in B-cell lymphomas. Cancer Sci 95:704-710,2004
58. Long CW. An account of the first use of sulphuric ether. Southern Med & Surg J 5:705-713,1849.
59. Lister J. On the antiseptic principle in the practice of surgery. The Lancet, 90:353-356,1867.
60. Asimov I. Asimov's biographical encyclopedia od science and technology.: The living stores of more than 1,000 great scientists from the Age of Greece to the Space Age, chronologically arranged. Garden City, NJ. Doubleday.
61. Flores J. Específico nuevamente descubierto en el reyno de Goatemala para la curacion the horrible mal de cancro y otros mas frecuentes, Cadiz, 1783.
62. Maunoir CT. Nouvelle méthode pour traiter le sarcocele sans extirper le testicule. Genève, 1820.
63. Boehm-Viswanathan T. Is angiogenesis inhibition the Holy Grail of cancer therapy? Curr Opin Oncol 12:89-94,2000.
64. Bennett H. On cancerous and cancroid growths, Edinburgh, 1849, p237.
65. Arnot J. Practical observations of the remedial efficacy of anaesthesic temperature in cancer, Lancet, Volume II, p257,1850
66. Zaffaroni N, Fiorentini G, De Giorgi U. Hyperthermia and hyposia: New developmentsin anticancer chemotherapy. Eur J Surg Oncol 27:340-342,2001.
67. Greve JW. Alternative techniques for the treatment of colon carcinoma metastases in the liver: current status in The Netherlands. Scand J Gastroenterol Suppl 234:77-81,2001.
68. Mala T, Edwin B, Gladhaug I, et al. Magnetic-resonance-guided percutaneous cryoablation of hepatic tumors. Eur J Surg 167:610-617,2001.
69. The Non-Hodgkin's Lymphoma Pathologic Classification Project. National Cancer Institute sponsored study of classifications of non-Hodgkin's lymphomas: summary and description of a working formulation for clinical usage. Cancer 49:2112-2135,1982
70. Harris NL, Jaffe ES, Kiebold J, el al. Lymphoma classification—from controversy to consensus: the REAL and WHO Classification of lymphoid neoplasms. Ann Oncol 11(suppl 1):S3-S10,2000.
71. Faguet GB. Chronic lymphocytic leukemia: An updated review. J Clin Oncol 12:1974-1990,1994.
72. Chronic lymphocytic leukemia: Advances in Molecular biology, Cytogenetics, Diagnosis, and Management. Ed Guy B. Faguet, Humana Press, 2003.
73. Age-adjusted incidence and U.S. deaths rates and 5-year relative survival rates (Table I-4), http://seer.cancer.gov/csr/1973_1999/overview/overview1.pdf

74. Venter JC, Adams MD, Meyers EW, et al. The sequence of the human genome. Science 291:1304-1351,2001.
75. International Human Genome Sequencing Consortium. Initial sequencing and analysis of the human genome. Nature 409:860-921,2001.
76. Kerem B, Rommens JM, Buchanan JA, et al. Identification of the cystic fibrosis gene: genetic analysis. Science 245:1073-80,1989
77. M. H. Polymeropoulos, C. Lavedan, E. Leroy, S. E. et al. Mutation in the α-Synuclein Gene Identified in Families with Parkinson's Disease. *Science* 276: 2045-2047,1997.
78. Watson James. The double Helix: A personal account of the discovery of the structure of DNA. Simon & Schuster; ISBN: 0684852799 1998. (1998)
79. Parshall G, Licking EF. James D. Watson JD, Francis Crick: Double-Teaming the Double Helix. US News & World Report, August 17, 1998, http:\\www.usnews.com/usnews/issue/980817/17dna.htm
80. Watson J, Crick F. A structure for deoxyribose nucleic acid. *Nature* 171:737,1953.
81. Sayre Anne. Rosalind Franklin and DNA. W.W. Norton & Company; ISBN: 0393320448 (2000)
82. http://www.ornl.gov/hgmis/posters/chromosome/
83. Sandberg A, Chen Z. Cytogenetic Analysis, *in* Hematologic Malignancies: Methods and Techniques, Ed Guy B Faguet, Human Press Inc., Totowa, New Jersey, 2001
84. Stadberg A, Chen Z. FISH analysis. *in* Hematologic Malignancies: Methods and Techniques, Ed Guy B Faguet, Human Press Inc., Totowa, New Jersey, 2001
85. Baudis M, Bentz M. Comparative genomic hybridization, *in* Hematologic Malignancies: Methods and Techniques, Ed Guy B Faguet, Human Press Inc., Totowa, New Jersey, 2001
86. Higenfeld E, Padilla-Nash H, Haas OA, et al. Spectral karyotyping (SKY) of hematologic malignancies, *in* Hematologic Malignancies: Methods and Techniques, Ed Guy B Faguet, Human Press Inc., Totowa, New Jersey, 2001
87. Mohr S, Leikauf GD, Keith G, et al. Microarrays as cancer keys: An array of possibilities. *J Clin Oncol* 20:3165-3175,2002.
88. Tsujimoto, Y., Gorham, J., Cossman, J., et al. The t(14;18) chromosome translocations involved in B-cell neoplasms result from mistakes in VDJ joining. Science, 229:1390-1393, 1985.
89. Moyzis RK, Buckingham JM, Cram LS, et al. A highly conserved repetitive DNA sequence (TTAGGG) present at the telomeres oh human chromosomes. Proc Natl Acad Sci USA 85:6622-6626,1988.
90. Shay JW and Bachetti S. A survey of telomerase activity in human cancer. Eur J Cancer 33:787-791,1997.
91. Futreal PA, Kspryk A, Birney E, et al. Cancer and Genomics. Nature 409:850-855,2001.
92. Hamblin TJ. Heterogeneous origin of the B-CLL cell, in Chronic Lymphocytic Leukemia: Advances in Molecular genetics, Biology, Diagnosis, and Management. Ed Guy B Faguet. The Humana Press, 2003.

93. Pignatelli M. Integrins, cadherins, and catenins: molecular cross-talk in cancer cells. J Pathol 186:1-21,1998.
94. Fidler I, Molecular biology of cancer: invasion and metastases. In: V.T.DeVita, S. Hellman, and S.A. Rosenberg (eds), Cancer principles and practice of oncology, Ed. 5, pp 135-152, New York: Lippincott-Raven, 1997.
95. Cronin K, Feuer E, Wesley M, et al. Current estimates for 5 and 10 year relative survival. Statistical Research and Applications Branch, NCI, Technical Report #2003-04.
96. Yoshida BA, Mitchell M, Sokoloff D, et al. Metastasis-suppressor genes: A review and perspective on an emerging field. Oncol Spectrums 2:166-192,2001.
97. Heimann R, Lan F, McBride R, et al. Separating favorable from unfavorable prognostic markers in breast cancer: the role of E-adherin. Nature 283:139-146,1980.
98. Heimann R, Ferguson DJ and Hellman S. The relationship between nm23, angiogenesis, and the metastatic proclivity of node-negative breast cancer. Cancer Res 58:2766-2771,1998.

PART   III

1. Arber E. Cell proliferation as a major risk for cancer: a concept of doubtful validity. Cancer Res 55: 3759-3762,1995.
2. Rosenberg SA. Identification of cancer antigens: impact on development of cancer immunotherapies. Cancer J Sci Am 6 (Suppl 3):S200-207, 2000
3. Reddy A, Kaelin G Jr. Using cancer genetics to guide the selection of anticancer drug targets. Curr Op Pharmacol 2:366-373,2002.
4. DeVita VT Jr, Serpick A. A combination chemotherapy in the treatment of Hodgkin's disease (HD). Proc Am Assoc Cancer Res 8:13,1967 (abstract).
5. Burnett FM. The concept of immunological surveillance, Prog Exp Tumor 13:1-27,1970.
6. Immune Surveillance. Eds RT Smith and M Landry. Academic Press, New York – London, 1970.
7. Mathé G, Amiel JL, Schwarzenberg L, et al. Active immunotherapy for acute lymphoblastic leukaemia. Lancet 1:697-699,1969.
8. Grasser I. Interferon and cancer: therapeutic prospects. Rev Eur Etud Clin Biol 15:23-7, 1970.
9. Amery WK, Spreafico F, Rojas AF, et al. Adjuvant treatment with levamisole in cancer: a review of experimental and clinical data. Cancer Treat Rev 4:167-94, 1977
10. Rosenberg SA, Lotze MT, Muul LM, Et al. Observations on the systemic administration of autologous lymphokine-activated killer cells and recombinant interleukin-2 to patients with metastatic cancer. N Engl J Med 313:1485-1492,1985.
11. Nelkin, D. Selling Science: how the press covers science and technology, W.H. Freeman & Company, New York, 1995.

12. Rosenberg SA. Progress in human tumour immunology and immunotherapy. Nature 411:380-384,2001.
13. Jager E, Knuth A. Clinical cancer vaccine trials. Current opinion in immunology 14:178-182,2002.
14. Blattner W. Epidemiology of HTLV-1 and associated diseases. (Blattner W, cd.). In Human retrovirology: IITLV-1. New York: Raven Press, 1990,251-265.
15. Gallo RC, Montagnier L. The chronology of AIDS research. Nature. 326:435-6,1987
16. Cesarman E, Chang Y, Moore PS, et al. Kaposi's sarcoma-associated herpesvirus-like DNA sequences in AIDS related body-cavity-based lymphomas. N Engl J Med 332:1186-1191,1995.
17. Einstein MH, Goldberg GL. Human papillovirus and cervical neoplasia. Cancer Invest 20:1080-1085,2002.
18. Blumberg BS, London WT. Hepatitis B virus: Pathogenesis and prevention of primary cancer of the liver. Cancer 50:2657-2665,1982.
19. Simonetti RG Camma C, Fiorello F, et al. Hepatitis C virus infection as a risk factor for hepatocellular carcinoma in patients with cirrhosis. Ann Int Med 116:97-102,1992.
20. Litter E, Baylis SA, Zeng Y, et al. Diagnosis of nasopharyngeal carcinoma by means of recombinant Epstein-Barr virus proteins. Lancet 337:685-689,1991.
21. Hematologic Malignancies: Methods and techniques. GB Faguet editor. Humana Press, 2001.
22. Brisco MJ. Quantifying residual leukemia by "clone-specific" polymerase chain reaction, in Hematologic Malignancies: Methods and techniques, GB Faguet editor, Humana Press, 2001.
23. Outcomes Working Group, Health Services Research Committee, America Society of Clinical Oncology. Outcomes of cancer treatment for technology assessment and cancer treatment guidelines. J Clin Oncol 14:671-679, 1996
24. Encyclopedia of the First World War: Deaths from gas attacks, http://www.spartacus.schoolnet.co.uk/FWWgasdeaths.htm
25. Kumbhaar EB, Kumbhaar HD. The blood and bone marrow in Yellow Cross Gas (Mustard Gas) poisoning: Changes produced in the bone marrow of fatal cases. J Med Res 40:497-507,1919.
26. Pappenheimer AM, Vance M. The effects of intravenous injections of Di-Chloroethylsulfide in rabbits, with special reference to its leukotoxic action. J Exp Med 31:71-95,1920.
27. Berenblum I. Experimental inhibition of tumor induction by mustard gas and other compounds. J Path Bact 40:549-558,1935.
28. Einhorn J. Nitrogen mustard: The origin oc chemotherapy for cancer. Int J Radiation Oncologt Biol Phys 11:1375-1378,1985.
29. Goodman LS, Wintrobe MM, Dameshek W, et al. Use of methyl-bis-(β-chloroethyl) amine hydrochloride and tris-(β-chloroethyl) amine hydrochloride for Hodgkin's disease, lymphosarcoma, leukemia, and certain allied and miscellaneous disorders. JAMA 132:126-132,1946.
30. Alexander SF. Medical report of the Bari Harbor Mustard casualties. The Military Surgeon 10:2-17,1947.

31. Jacobson LO, Spurr CL, Barron ES, et al. Studies of the effect of methyl methyl-bis-(β-chloroethyl) amine hydrochloride on neoplastic diseases and allied disorders of the hemopoietic system. JAMA 132:263,1946.

32. Karnofsky DA, Carver LF, Rhoads CF et al. An evaluation of methyl-bis-(β-chloroethyl) amine hydrochloride (nitrogen mustards) in the treatment of lymphomas, leukemias, and allied diseases, in Moulton FR (ed): Approach to cancer chemotherapy. Washington DC, AAAS, 1947.

33. Rhoads CP. Report on a cooperative study of nitrogen mustard (HN2) therapy of neoplastic disease. Trans Assoc Am Physicians 60, 1947.

34. Goodman LS, Wintrobe MM, Dameshek W, et al. Nitrogen mustard therapy. JAMA 132:126-132,1946.

35. Woods DD. The relation of p-aminobenzoic acid to the mechanism of action of sulfaniamide. Br J Exp Pathol 21:74,1940.

36. Fildes P. A rational approach to research in chemotherapy. Lancet 1:995,1940.

37. Seeger DR, Smith JM Fr, Hultquist ME. Antagonist for pteroylglutamic acid. J Am Chem Soc 69:2567,1947.

38. Seeger DR, Cosulich DB, Smith JM Jr, et al. Analogs of pteroylglutamic acid III. 4-amino derivatives. J Am Chem Soc 71:1753,1949.

39. Farber S, Diamond LK, Mercer RD et al. Temporary remissions in acute leukemia in children produced by the folic acid antagonist, 4-aminopteroylglutamic acid (Aminopterin). N Engl J Med 238:787,1948.

40. Hertz R, Lewis J, Lipsett M. Five years experience with chemotherapy of metastatic choriocarcinoma and related trophoblastic tumors in women. Am J Obstet Gynecol 1961;82:631.59.

41. Burchenal JH, Murphy ML, Ellison RR, et al. Clinical evaluation of a new antimetabolite, 6-mercaptopurine, in the treatment of leukemia and allied diseases. Blood 8:965,1953.

42. Murphy ML, Tan TC, Ellison RR, et al. Clinical evaluation of chloroquine and thioguanine. Proc Am Assoc Cancer Res 2:36,1955 (abstract).

43. Cited in Groopman V. The thirty year war: Have we being fighting cancer the wrong way? The New Yorker, June 4th, 2001, p53.

44. Drug discovery at the National Institute of Cancer, March 1, 2002, http://newscenter.cancer.gov/pressreleases/discovery.html

45. Bainbridge WS. The cancer problem. New York, MacMillan, 1914.

46. Sikora K, Advani S, Koroltchouk V, et al. Essential drugs for cancer therapy: A World Health Organization Consultation. Annals Oncol 10:385-390,1999 (revised list posted in April 2003 http://mednet3.int/Eml/disease_factsheet.asp?diseaseId=530).

47. Woglom WH. General review of cancer therapy, in Moulton FR (ed): Approaches to tumor chemotherapy. Washington, DC AAAS, 1947, pg1.

48. Druker BJ, Talpaz M, Resta DJ, et al, Efficacy and safety of a specific inhibitor of the BCR-ABL tyrosine kinase in chronic myeloid leukemia. N Engl J Med 344:1031-1037,2001.

49. Tannock I. Cell kinetics and chemotherapy: a critical review. Cancer Treat Rep 62:1117-1133,1978.

50. Skipper HE. Historic milestones in cancer biology: a few that are important to cancer treatment (revisited). Semin Oncol 6:506-514,1979.
51. Mendelsohn ML. The growth fraction: a new concept applied to tumors. Science 132:1496,1960.
52. Goldie JH, Coldman AJ. A mathematical model for relating the drug sensitivity of tumors to their spontaneous mutations rate. Cancer Treat Rep 63:1727-1733,1979.
53. Laird AK.. Dynamics of growth in tumors and normal organisms, Natl Cancer Inst Monogr 30:15-281969.
54. Bonadonna G, Rossi A, Valagussa BS. Adjuvant CMF in operable breast cancer: ten years later. Wolrd J Surg 5:95-115,1985.
55. Jemal A, Thomas A, Murray T, et al. Cancer statistics, 2002.CA Cancer J Clin 52:23-47,2002.
56. Breathnach O, Freidlin B, Conley B, et al. Twenty-two years of phase III trials for patients with advanced non-small-cell lung cancer: sobering results. J Clin Oncol 19:1734-1742, 2000.
57. Karnofsky DA, Abelmann WH, Craver LF, et al. The use of nitrogen mustards in the palliative treatment of carcinoma. Cancer 634-656, 1948.
58. Kennedy BJ. The snail's pace of lung carcinoma chemotherapy. Cancer 82:801-803,1998.
59. Non-small cell lung cancer collaborative group. Chemotherapy for non-small cell lung cancer (Cochrane Review), In: The Cochrane Library, Issue 2, 2002. Oxford: Update Software.
60. Schiller J, Harrington D, Belani CP, et al. Comparison of four chemotherapy regimens for advanced non-small-cell lung cancer. N Engl J Med 346:92-8,2002.
61. Evans WK. The cost and cost-effectiveness of treating non-small cell lung cancer. Oncology Spectrums 3:35-41,2002.
62. Martin DS, Gelhorn A. Combinations of chemical compounds in experimental cancer chemotherapy. Cancer Res 11:35,1951.
63. Skipper HE. Nucleotide metabolism and cancer chemotherapy, in Rebuck JW, Bethell FH, Monto RW (eds): The Leukemias: Etiology, Pathophysiology, and Treatment. New York, Academic 1957, p541.
64. Freireich EJ, Karon M, Frei E III. Quadruple combination therapy (VAMP) for acute lymphoblastic leukemia of childhood. Proc Am Assoc Cancer Res 5:20,1964 (abstract).
65. DeVita VT Jr, Serpick A. Combination chemotherapy in the treatment of advanced Hodgkin's disease (HD). Proc Am Assoc Cancer Res 8:13,1967 (Abstract)
66. Devita VT Jr, Simon RM, Hubbard SM et al. Curability of advanced Hodgkin's disease with chemotherapy: Long-term followu-up of MOPP-treated patients at the National Cancer Institute (NCI). Ann Intern Med. 92:586-595,1980.
67. Donohue JP, Einhorn LH, Perez JM. Improved management of non-seminomatous testis tumors. Cancer 42:2903-8,1978.
68. Surbone A and DeVita VT Jr. Dose intensity. The neglected variable in clinical trials. Ann NY Acad Sci 698:279-288,1993.

69. Hryaiuk WA, Figueredo A, Goodyear M. Application of dose intensity to problems in chemotherapy of breast and colon cancer. Semin Oncol 1987;14(suppl 4)3-11.
70. Waxman S, Anderson KC. History of the development of arsenic derivatives in cancer therapy. The Oncologist 6:3-10,2001.
71. Aublanc JB. Dissertations sur le cancer. Paris 1803, pg 40.
72. Stephenson J. Bone marrow/Stem cells: No edge in breast cancer. JAMA 281:1641-1642,1999.
73. Stadtmauer EA, O'Neil A, Goldstein LJ, et al. Conventional-dose chemotherapy compared with high-dose chemotherapy plus autologous hematopoietic stem-cell transplantation for metastatic breast cancer. Philadelphia Bone Marrow Transplant Group. N Engl J Med 342:1069-1076,2000.
74. Editorial. Retraction. J Clin Oncol 2001 Jun 1;19(11):2973
75. Farquhar C, Basser R, Marjoribanks J, et al.. High dose chemotherapy and autologous bone marrow or stem cell transplantation versus conventional chemotherapy for women with early poor prognosis breast cancer (Cochrane Review). In: The Cochrane Library, Issue e, 2004. Chichester, UK: John Wiley & Sons, ltd.
76. Kyle RA. The role of high-dose chemotherapy in the treatment of multiple myeloma: a controversy. Ann Oncol 11(Suppl 1):55-58,2000.
77. Kolb HJ, Socie G, Duell T, et al. Malignant neoplasms in long-term survivors of bone marrow transplantation. Late Effects Working Party of the European Cooperative Group for Blood and Marrow Transplantation and the European Late Effect Project Group. Ann Intern Med 131:738-744,1999.
78. Perry MC. The chemotherapy source book. Williams and Wilkins, Baltimore, MD, 1992.
79. Sporn MB. The war on cancer. The lancet 347:1377-1381,1996.
80. DeVita VT. The War on cancer has a birthday, and a present. J Clin Oncol 15:867-869,1997.
81. Special Report: Measurement of Progress Against Cancer. Extramural Committee to Assess Measures of Progress Against Cancer. J Natl Cancer Inst 82:825-835,1990.
82. Edwards, BK, Howe HL, Ries LAG, et al. Annual Report to the Nation on the status of cancer, 1973-1999, featuring implications of age and aging on U.S. cancer burden. Cancer 94: 2766-2792,2002.
83. Andersen LD, Remington P, Trentham-Dietz A, et al. Assessing a decade of progress in cancer control. The Oncologist 7:200-204,2002.
84. Weir HK, Thun MJ, Hankey BF, et al. The Annual Report to the Nation on the Status of Cancer 1975-2000, Featuring the Use of Surveillance Data for Cancer Prevention and Control. J. Natl. Cancer Inst. 95:1276-1299,2003.
85. Kiebert G, Wait S, Beernhard J, et al. Practice and Policy of measuring quality of life and health economics in cancer trials: A survey among co-operative trial groups. Qual Life Res. 9:1073-1080,2000.
86. Kuenstner S, Langelotz C, Budach V, et al. The comparability of quality of life scores. a multitrait multimethod analysis of the EORTC QLQ-C30, SF-36 and FLIC questionnaires. Eur J Cancer 38:339-48,2002.

87. Slevin ML, Stubbs L, Plant HJ, et al. Attitudes to chemotherapy: comparing views of patients with cancer with those of doctors, nurses, and general public. Br Med J 300:1458-1460,1990.
88. Schipper H, Goh CR, Wang TL. Shifting the cancer paradigm: Must we kill to cure? J Clin Oncol 13:801-805,1995.

PART IV

1. Bailar JC 3rd, Smith EM. Progress against cancer? N Engl J Med. 314:1226-1232,1986
2. Bailar JC 3rd, Gornik HL. Cancer undefeated. N Engl J Med. 336:1569-1574,1997
3. Sporn MB. The war on cancer. The lancet 347:1377-1381,1996.
4. Epstein, SS The Politics of Cancer Revisited. East Ridge Press, Hankins, NY, 1998.
5. *Cox, Patrick: Ralph W. Yarborough, the People's Senator* University of Texas Press. ISBN: 029271243X, January 2002
6. Farber S, Diamond LK, Mercer RD et al. Temporary remissions in acute leukemia in children produced by the folic acid antagonist, 4-aminopteroylglutamic acid (Aminopterin). N Engl J Med 238:787,1948
7. Garb S. Cure for Cancer A National Goal. Springer, N.Y. 1968.
8. Cited in Groopman J. The thirty year war: Have we being fighting cancer the wrong way? The New Yorker, June 4th, 2001, p53.
9. The Richard Nixon Library and Birthplace, http://nixonfoundation.org/Research_Center/1971_pdf_files/1971_0026.pdf
10. http://www.nci.nih.gov/aboutnci/org.htm
11. A Plan and Budget Proposal for Fiscal Year 2005. NIH Publication No 03-5446, Oct 2003.
12. http://cancernet.nci.nih.gov/trialsrch.shtml
13. Louis, PCA. Essays in Clinical Instruction. London, UK: P. Martin; 1834.
14. Louis PCA. Researches into the effects of blood-letting in some inflammatory diseases and on the influence of tartarized antimony and vessication in pneumonitis. Am J Med Sci 1836;18:102-111.
15. DeVita VT Jr, Serpick A. Combination chemotherapy in the treatment of advanced Hodgkin's disease (HD). Proc Am Assoc Cancer Res 8:13,1967 (Abstract)
16. Selen M. Theory and practice of clinical trials. E-Medicine, http://www.cancer.org
17. Faguet GB, Davis HC: Regression analysis in medical research. Southern Med. J. 77:722-725, 1984.
18. Breathnach O, Freidlin B, Conley B, et al. Twenty-two years of phase III trials for patients with advanced non-small-cell lung cancer: sobering results. J Clin Oncol 19:1734-1742, 2000.
19. EORTC's "Open protocols", http://www.eortc.be/
20. Fisher B, Costantino JP, Wickerham DL, et al. Tamoxifen for prevention of breast cancer: Report of the National Surgical Adjuvant

Breast and Bowel Project P-1 Study. J Natl Cancer Inst 90:1371-1388,1998.

21. Levine M, Moutquin JM, Walton R, et al; Canadian Task Force on Preventive Health Care and the Canadian Breast Cancer Initiative's Steering Committee on Clinical Practice Guidelines for the Care and Treatment of Breast Cancer Chemoprevention of breast cancer. A joint guideline from the Canadian Task Force on Preventive Health Care and the Canadian Breast Cancer Initiative's Steering Committee on Clinical Practice Guidelines for the Care and Treatment of Breast Cancer. Can Med Assoc J 164:1681-90,2001

22. http://bcra.nci.nih.gov/brc/

23. Powles T, Eeles R, Ashley S, et al. Interim analysis of the incidence of breast cancer in the Royal Marsden Hospital tamoxifen randomized chemoprevention trial. Lancet 352:98-101,1998.

24. Veronesi U, Maisonneuve P, Sacchini V, et al. Tamoxifen for breast cancer among hysterectomised women. Lancet 359:1122-1124,2002.

25. Future possibilities in the prevention of breast cancer. Breast cancer prevention trials Breast Cancer Res 2:258-263,2000.

26. Study of Tamoxifen and Raloxifene (STAR) for the Prevention of Breast Cancer, http://www.cancer.gov/clinicaltrials/view_clinicaltrials.aspx?version=patient&cdrid=67081

27. Editorials. Peer review: reform or revolution. Br Med J 315:759-760,1997.

28. Public library of science, http://www.publiclibraryofscience.org/

29. Editorials. Measuring the social impact of research. Br Med J 323:528,2001.

30. Eisenhofer G. Scientific productivity: Waning importance for career development of today's scientists?, http://his.com/~graeme/pandp.html

31. National Surgical Adjuvant Breast and Bowel Project, available online at http://www.nsabp.pitt.edu/

32. Southwest Oncology Group, http://swog.org/visitors/WhatWedo.asp

33. Grabowski H, Vernon J. Returns to R&D on new drug introductions in the 1980s. J Health Econ 13:383-406,1994.

34. Pharmaceutical research and manufacturers of America, http://www.phrma.org/

35. Djulbegovic B, Lacevic M, Cantor A, et al. The uncertainty principle and industry-sponsored research Lancet 356:635-638,2000.

36. Blumenthal D, Campbell EG, Anderson MS, et al. Withholding research results in academic life science: Evidence from a national survey of faculty JAMA 277:1224-1228,1997.

37. Schulman KA, Seils DM, Timbie JW, et al. A national survey of provisions in clinical-trial agreements between medical schools and industry sponsors. N Engl J Med 347:1335-1341,2002.

38. Science-Scope: Strength in numbers. Science 293:1969,2001

39. 39 Carlsson M. Cancer patients seeking information from sources outside the health care system. Support Care Cancer 8:453-457,2000.

40. Pentz RD, Flamm AL, Sugarman J, et al. Study of the media's potential influence on prospective research participants' understanding of and

motivations for participation in a high-profile phase I trial. J Clin Oncol. 20:3785-91,2002.

41. MacDonald MM, Hoffman-Goetz L. A retrospective study of the accuracy of cancer information in Ontario daily newspapers. Can J Public Health 93:142-145,2002.
42. Medicine in the Media: The Challenge of Reporting on Medical Research Symposium. Rockville, MD, June 23-25,2002.
43. Editorials. Have we lost are way? The Lancet 341:343-344,1993.
44. The American Board of Internal Medicine, http://www.abim.org
45. http://www.sciencekomm.at/journals/medicine/onco.html
46. American Society of Clinical Oncology, http://www.asco.org/
47. America Society of Hematology, http://www.hematology.org/
48. Varmus H. Disease-specific estimates of direct and indirect costs of illness and NIH support. Bethesda, MD: Department of Health and Human Services, National Institutes of Health, Office of the Director, September 1997.
49. Johnson DH. Evolution of cisplatin-based chemotherapy in non-small cell lung cancer: a historical perspective and the eastern cooperative oncology group experience. Chest 117:133S-137S,2000.
50. Coiffier B, Lepage E, Brière J, et al. CHOP chemotherapy plus rituximab compared with CHOP alone in elderly patients with diffuse large- B-cell lymphoma. N Engl J Med 346:235-242,2002.
51. Cheson BD. CHOP plus Rituximab – Balancing facts and opinion.
52. Emanuel EJ, Dubler NN. Preserving the physician-patient relationship in the era of managed care. JAMA 273:323-329,1995.
53. Council of Ethical and Judicial Affairs, American Medical Association: Ethical issues in managed care. JAMA 273:330-335,1995.
54. Gray BH. The profit motive and patient care: The changing accountability of doctors and hospitals. Cambridge, MA Harvard University,1991.
55. Hillman BJ, Joseph CA, Mabry MR, et al. Frequency and costs of diagnostic imaging in office practice - A comparison to self-referring and radiologist-referring physicians. New Engl J Med 327:1604-1608,1990.
56. Kurowski B. Six key challenges in oncology disease management. Dis Manag 1:99,1998.
57. Smyth A. Reimbursement issues for the oncologist. Oncol Reimbursement 1:1-4,1993.
58. Smith TJ, Girtman J, Riggins J. Why academic Divisions of Hematology/Oncology are in trouble and some suggestions for resolution. J Clin Oncol 19:260-264,2001.
59. Medical Group Management Association: Academic Practice Faculty Compensation and Production survey. 1999 Report based on 1998 Data. Medical Group Management Association. Englewood Co. 1000, pp 28-31.
60. Halbert RJ, Zaher C, Wade S, et al. Outpatient cancer drug costgs: charges, drivers, and the future. Cancer 94:1142-1150,2002.
61. Bennett CL, Bishop MR, Tallman MS, et al. The association between physician reimbursement in the US and use of hematopoietic colony stimulation factors as adjunct therapy for older patients with acute

myeloid leukemia: results from the 1997 American Society of Clinical Oncology survey. Health Services Research Committee of the American Society of Clinical Oncology. Ann Oncol 11:1355-1359,1999.

62. Use of hematopoietic colony-stimulation factors: the American Society of Clinical Oncology survey. The Health Services Research Committee of the American Society of Clinical Oncology. J Clin Oncol 9:2511-2520,1996.

63. Ozer H. American Society of Clinical Oncology guidelines for the use of hematopoietic colony-stimulating factors. Curr Opin Hematol 3:3-10,1996.

64. Cavo M, Benni M, Ronconi S, et al. Melphalan-prednisone versus alternating combination VAD/MP or VND/MP as primary therapy for multiple myeloma: final analysis of a randomized clinical study. Haematologica. 87:934-42,2002.

65. McLaughlin P, Grillo-Lopez AJ, Link BK, et al. Rituximab chimeric anti-CD20

66. monoclonal antibody therapy for relapsed indolent lymphoma: Half of patients respond to a four-dose treatment program. J Clin Oncol 16:2825-2833,1998.

67. Genentech,   Rituxan   sales, http://www.com/gene/ir/financials/historical/rituxan.jsp

68. Stephenson J. Bone marrow/Stem cells: No edge in breast cancer. JAMA 281:1641-1642,1999.

69. Stadtmauer EA, O'Neill A, Goldstein LJ, et al. Conventional-dose chemotherapy compared with high-dose chemotherapy plus autologous hematopoietic stem-cell transplantation for metastatic breast cancer. Philadelphia Bone Marrow Transplant Group. N Engl J Med 342:1069-1076,2000.

70. Faguet GB. Chronic lymphocytic leukemia: An updated review. J Clin Oncol 12:1974-1990,1994.

71. Chronic Lymphocytic Leukemia: Advances in Molecular genetics, Biology, Diagnosis, and Management, Ed Guy B Faguet, Humana Press, Inc. Totowa, N J, 2003

72. Dighiero G. Guidelines for the clinical management of chronic lymphocytic leukemia in Chronic Lymphocytic Leukemia: Advances in Molecular genetics, Biology, Diagnosis, and Management, Ed Guy B Faguet, Humana Press, Inc. Totowa, NJ, 2003.

73. Morrison VA, Rai KR, Peterson BL, et al. Impact of therapy with chlorambucil, fludarabine, or fludarabine plus chlorambucil on infections in patients with chronic lymphocytic leukemia: Intergroup Study Cancer and Leukemia Group B 9011. J Clin Oncol. 19:3611-3621,2001.

74. Kalil N, Cheson BD. Management of chronic lymphocytic leukemia. Drugs   Aging   16:9-27,2000. 74. Grant T. Doctor's Work: The legacy of Sir William Osler. Firefly Books. 2003.

75. http://www.schering.de/eng/irf.html?/eng/investorrelationsforum/public ations/annualreports/annualreport2001/

76. Kübler-Ross E. On death and dying. Touchstone, New York, NY, 1997.

77. Jenkins V, Fallowfield L, Saul J. Information needs of patients with cancer: results from a large study in UK cancer centers. Br J Cancer 84:48-51,2001.
78. Parker PA, Baile WF, de Moor C, et al. Breaking bad news about cancer" patients' preferences for communications. J Clin Oncol 19:2049-2056,2001.
79. Loge JH, Kaasa S, Hytten K. Disclosing the cancer diagnosis: the patients' experiences. Eur J Cancer 33:878-882,1997.
80. Bruera E, Neumann CM, Mazzocato C, et al. Attitudes and beliefs of palliative care physicians regarding communication s with terminally ill cancer patients. Palliat Med 14:287-298,2000.
81. Grassi L, Giraldi T Messina EG, et al. Physicians attitudes to and problems with truth-telling to cancer patients. Support Care Cancer 8:40-50,2000.
82. Fallowfield LJ, Jenkins VA, Beveridge HA. Truth may hurt but deceit hurts more: communication in palliative care. Palliat Med 16:297-302,2002.
83. Kaplowitz SA, Campo S, Chiu WT. Cancer patients' desires for communication of prognosis information. Health Commun 14:221-41,2002.
84. The National Commission for the Protection of Human Subjects of Biomedical and Behavioral Research, "The Belmont Report: Ethical Principles and Guidelines for the Protection of Human Subjects of Research." April 18, 1979. Department of Health and Human Services, Publication No. (OS) 780013 and No. (OS) 78-0014, Superintendent of Documents, U.S. Government Printing Office, Washington, D.C. 20402.
85. Owen E. Time Daily "Tuskegee Apology: Clinton makes amends to victims of Tuskegee study, May 16, 1997, http://www.pathfinder.com/@@NwQDWgcAlAFuYgO5/time
86. Department of Energy. Advisory Committee on Human Radiation Experiments - Final Report. Superintendent of Documents U.S. Government Printing Office. Washington, D.C. 20402, June 1998, http://nattie.eh.doe.gov/systems/hrad/report.html
87. Lalli AN. Arguments for Informed Consent Without Waivers | or Exceptions: An Analysis of Common Rule by September, 1997, http://pw2.netcom.com/~alalli/BillSite_analysis/paper_web.html
88. Lalli AN. Letter to: Secretary Donna E. Shalala | Dept. Health and Human Services. June 06, 2000, http://pw2.netcom.com/~alalli/BillSite_analysis/shalala_letter.html
89. Leighl N, Gattleari M, Butow P, et al. Discussing adjuvant cancer therapy. J Clin Oncol 19:1768-1778,2001.
90. Yardley SJ, Davis CL, Sheldon F. Receiving a diagnosis of lung cancer: patients' interpretations, perceptions and perspectives. Palliat Med 15:379-86,2001
91. Fred Hutchinson Cancer Research Center, finds violations of federal law, http://www.fda.gov/foi/warning_letters/g2083d.pdf to Dr. Dana Matthews, Dec. 31, 2001.
92. Cook-Deegan RM. Cloning human beings, http://www.bioethics.georgetown.edu/nbac/pubs/cloning2/cc8.pdf

93. Clinical research comes under scrutiny. The Lancer 2:588,2001.
94. Nakajima K, Bidaillon D. Communication issues in the managed care environment. Forum 17:6-9,1996.
95. Slevin ML, Stubbs L, Plant HJ, et al. Attitudes to chemotherapy: comparing views of patients with cancer with those of doctors, nurses, and general public. Br Med J 300:1458-1460,1990.
96. Carlsson M. Cancer patients seeking information from sources outside the health care system. Support Care Cancer 8:453-457,2000.
97. Cassileth BR, Zupkis RV, Sutton-Smith K, et al. Information and participation preferences among cancer patients. Ann Intern Med 92:832-836,1980.
98. Gattellari M, Butow PN, Tattersall MH. Informed consent: what did the doctor say? Lancet. 353:1713,1999.
99. Coulter A. Partnerships with patients: the pros and cons of shared clinical decision making. J Health Service Res Policy 2:112-121,1997.
100. Charles C, Whelam T, Gafni A. What do we mean by partnership in making decisions about treatment? Br Med J 319:780-782,1999.
101. Degner LF, Krsitjanson LJ, Bowman D, et al. Information needs and decisional preferences in women with breast cancer. JAMA 277:1485-1492,1997.
102. Siminoff IA, Fetting JH, Abeloff MD. Doctor-patient communications about breast cancer adjuvant therapy. J Clin Oncol 7:1192-1200,1989.
103. O'Connor AM, Fiset V, DeGrasse C, et al. Decision aids for patients considering options affecting cancer outcomes: evidence of efficacy and policy implications. J Natl Cancer Inst Monogr 25:67-80,1999.
104. NCI's simplified informed consent, http://www.nci.nih.gov/clinical_trials/doc_header.aspx?viewid=5fca4dc5-b6a7-4272-be96-b489f23022e5&docid=3fccc228-0fe5-4d3a-a3b7-5eb825724da4
105. Ahmedin J, Thomas A, Murray T, et al. Facts and Figures, 2002. CA Cancer J Clin 52:23-47,2002
106. Blackhall LJ. Must we always use CPR? N Engl J Med 317:1281-1285,1987.
107. Paris JJ, Crone RK, Reardon F. Physicians' refusal of requested treatment. N Engl J Med 322:1012-1015,1990.
108. Leadbetter R. Danaus. Encyclopedia Mythica, http://www.pantheon.org/mythica.html
109. Council on Ethical and Judicial Affairs, Code of Medical Ethics, Chicago, IL: American Medical Association, 1998-1999.
110. Caplan AL. Odds and ends: trust and the debate over medical futility. Ann Intern Med 125:688-689,1996.
111. Schneiderman LJ, Jecker NS, Jonsen AR. Medical futility: Response to critics. Ann Inter Med 125:669-674,1996.
112. Scneiderman LJ, Jecker NS, Jonsen AR. Medical futility: its meaning and ethical implications. Ann Intern Med 112:949-954,1990.
113. Kite S, Wilkinson S. Beyond futility: to what extent is the concept of futility useful in clinical decision-making about CPR?. Lancet Oncol 3:638-642,2002.
114. Berry DA, Broadwater G, Klein JP, et al. High-dose versus standard chemotherapy in metastatic breast cancer: comparison of Cancer and

Leukemia Group B trials with data from the Autologous Blood and Marrow Transplant Registry. J Clin Oncol 20:743-750,2002.

115. Powles TJ, Coombes RC, Smith IE, et al. Failure of chemotherapy to prolong survival in a group of patients with metastatic breast cancer. Lancet 1:580-582,1980.

116. Califano, JA Jr., Physician-Assisted Living, America, November 14, 1998, pp.10-12.

117. Locational Information: The Routes of Santiago de Compostela in France, http://whc.unesco.org/sites/868-loc.htm

118. Saunders C. The evolution of hospices. Free inquiry. Winter 1991/92:19-23.

119. A controlled trial to improve care for seriously ill hospitalized patients. The Study to Understand Prognoses and Preferences for Outcomes and Risks of Treatments (SUPPPORT). The SUPPORT Principal Investigators. JAMA 1995;274:1591-1598.

120. World Health Organization. Cancer pain relief and palliative care. Geneva, Switzerland: World Health Organization; 1990:11-12.

PART V

1. Kuhn, TS. The Structure of Scientific Revolutions, University of Chicago Press, Chicago, 1962.

2. 2001 Cancer Progress Report, http://progressreport.cancer.gov/

3. Fisher B , Costantino JP, Wickerham DL, et al. Tamoxifen for prevention of breast cancer: Report of the National Surgical Adjuvant Breast and Bowel Project P-1 Study. J Nat Cancer Institute 90:1371-1388,1998.

4. History of tobacco, http://www.tobacco.org/History/Tobacco_History.html

5. National Vital Statistics Report, Vol 49 No. 11, October 12, 2001.

6. Jemal A, Thomas A, Murray T, et al. Cancer statistics, 2002. CA: A cancer journal for clinicians. 52:23-47,2002.

7. Nelson DE, Kirkendall RS, Lawton RL, et al. Surveillance for smoking-attributable mortality and years of potential life lost, by state - United States, 1990. Morbidity and Mortality Weekly Report 43(1):1-8,1994.

8. Newcomb PA, Carbone PP, The health consequences of smoking: cancer. In: Fiore MC, Ed. Cigarette Smoking: A Clinical Guide to Assessment and Treatment. Philadelphia, PA: WB Saunders Co; 1992: 305-331, Medical Clinics of North America.

9. Peto R, Lopez, A.D., Boreham, J., et al. Mortality from smoking in developed countries, 1950-2000: Indirect estimates from national vital statistics. New York, NY: Oxford University Press, 1994.

10. The World Health Report, 1999 Making a Difference. World Health Organization.

11. Tobacco and related Health-R&D approach. Report to R&D Committee of the Philip Morris Inc, by Dr. H. Wakeman. New York Office, November 15, 1961.

12. Ontario Task force on the primary prevention of cancer: Recommendations for the primary prevention of cancer. Toronto, Canada: Queen's printer for Ontario, 1995.
13. Knekt P, Hakama M, Jarvinen R, et al. Smoking and risk of colorectal cancer. Br J Cancer 78:136-139,1998.
14. Wingo PA, Lynn AG, Ries MS, et al: Annual report to the nation on the status of cancer, 1973-1996, with a special section on lung cancer and tobacco smoking. J Natl Cancer Inst 91:675-690,1999.
15. Greelee RT, Hill-Harmon MB, Murray T, et al. Cancer statistics, 2001 CA: A cancer journal for clinicians 51:15-27,2001.
16. A six-month investigation by NOW with Bill Moyers, THE NATION, and the Center for Investigative Reporting, aired by PBS on April 19,2002, http://www.pbs.org/now/indepth/041902_smuggling.html
17. Tobacco use in the US, 1990-1999, http://intouchlive.com/journals/oncology/o0007f.htm (extracted from Morbidity and Mortality Weekly Report 48:986-993,1999.
18. Framework Convention Alliance: Building support of global tobacco control. http://fctc.org/sign_rat/signed.shtml
19. Grossman M and Chaloupka FJ. Cigarette taxes: The straw to break the camel's back. Public Health Rep 112:290-297,1997.
20. Lung Association Report Reviews Tobacco Laws enacted in 2001, Feb 14, 2002, http://longusa.org/press/tobacco/tobacco_021402html
21. Leigh J, Berry G, de Klerk NH, et al. Asbestos-related lung cancer: apportionment of causation and damages to asbestos and tobacco smoke. Asbestos Pathenogenesis and Litigation. G. A. Peters and B. J. Peters. Charlottesville, VA, Michie. 13: pp 141-166 (1996)
22. Blattner W. Epidemiology of HTLV-1 and associated diseases. (Blattner W, ed.). In Human retrovirology: HTLV-1. New York: Raven Press, pp 251-265 (1990)
23. Litter E, Baylis SA, Zeng Y, et al. Diagnosis of nasopharyngeal carcinoma by means of recombinant Epstein-Barr virus proteins. Lancet 337:685-689,1991.
24. Einstein MH, Goldberg GL. Human papillovirus and cervical neoplasia. Cancer Invest 20:1080-1085,2002.
25. Blumberg BS, London WT. Hepatitis B virus: Pathogenesis and prevention of primary cancer of the liver. Cancer 50:2657-2665,1982.
26. Simonetti RG, Camma C, Fiorello F, et al. Hepatitis C virus infection as a risk factor for hepatocellular carcinoma in patients with cirrhosis: A case-control study. Ann Int Med 116:97-102,1992
27. Hausen H. Viral oncogenesis, in Microbes and malignancy. Infection as a cause of human cancer. I Parmont, Ed. New York: Oxford University Press, 1999 pp 107-130.
28. Caselmann W. Pathogenesis of hepatocellular carcinoma. Digestion 59:60-63,1998.
29. The World Cancer Report, Ed Kleihues P, Stewart BW. Press release 3 April, 2003, http://www.who.int/mediacentre/releases/2003/pr27/en/
30. Blumberg BS, Blumberg BS, Larouze B. et al. The relation of infection with hepatitis B agent to primary hepatic carcinoma. Am J Pathol 81:669-682,1975.

31. Tsukuma H, Hiyama T, Tanaka S, et al. Risk factors for hepatocellular carcinoma among patients with chronic liver disease. N Engl J Med. 328:1797-801,1993.
32. Bosch FX, Ribes J, Borras J, et al. Epidemiology of primary liver cancer. Sem Liver Dis 19:271-285,1999.
33. 33 Bruix J, Barrera JM, Calvet X, et al. Prevalence of antibodies to hepatitis C virus in Spanish patients with hepatocarcinoma and hepatic cirrhosis. Lancet 2:1004-1006,1989.
34. Parkin M, Muir CS, Wheelan SL, et al., eds. Cancer Incidence in Five Continents, vol. VI (IARC Scientific Publication No 120). Lyon: International Agency for Research on Cancer, 1992
35. National Center for Infectious Diseases, Center for Disease Control and Prevention, http://www.cdc.gov/ncidod/diseases/hepatitis/index.htm
36. Monto A, Wright TH. The epidemiology and prevention of hepatocellular carcinoma. Semin Oncol 28:441-449,2001.
37. 4. Jemal A, Tiwari RC, Murray T, et al. Cancer Facts & Figures 2004. CA Cancer J Clin 2004; 54:8-29. http://www.cancer.org/docroot/STT/stt_0.asp
38. Yoshizama H. Hepatocellular carcinoma associated with hepatitis C virus infection in Japan: projection to other countries in the foreseeable future. Oncology 62:8-17,2001.
39. Achievements in Public Health, 1900-1999; Impact of vaccines universally recommended for children – United States, 1900-1998. MMWR, April 2, 1999; vol 48, No 12.
40. World Health. The magazine of the WHO, May 1980.
41. Chang MH, Chen CJ, Lai MS, et al. Universal hepatitis B vaccination in Taiwan and the incidence of hepatocellular carcinoma in children. N Engl J Med 336:1855-1859,1997.
42. Schiller JT, Lowy DR: Papillomavirus-like particle based vaccines: cervical cancer and beyond. Expert Opin Biol Ther. 1: 571-581, 2001.
43. Koutsky LA, Ault KA, Wheeler CW, et al. A controlled trial of a human papillomavirus type 16 vaccine. N Engl J Med 347:1645-1651,2002.
44. Harper DM, Franco EL, Wheeler C., et al. Efficacy of a bivalent L1 virus-like particle vaccine in prevention of infection with human papillomavirus types 16 and 18 in young women: a randomised controlled trial. Lancet 364:1757-1765,2004.
45. Malcolm Gladwell. The Picture Problem: Mammography, air power, and the limits of looking. The New Yorker, Dec 13, 2004.
46. Smith RA, Mettlin CJ, Davis KJ, et al. American Cancer Society guidelines for the early detection of cancer. CA Cancer J Clin 50:34-49,2000.
47. Potosky AL, Kessler L, Gridley G, et al. Rise in prostatic cancer incidence associated with increased use of transurethral resection. J NCI 82:1624-1628,1990.
48. SEER Cancer Statistics Review, 1973-1999, http://seer.cancer.gov/csr/1973_1999/lung.pdf
49. McNeal JE Bostwick DG, Kindrachuk RA, et al. Patterns of progression in prostate cancer. Lancet 8472,60-63,1986.

50. Chodak GW, Shoenberg HW. Early detection of prostate cancer by routine screening. JAMA 252:3261-3264,1984.
51. Wajsman Z, Chu TM: Detection and diagnosis of prostate cancer. In: Murphy GP ed. Prostatic cancer. Littleton Mass. 1987, pp94-99.
52. Richert-Boe KE, Humphrey LL, Glass AG, et al. Screening digital rectal examination and prostate cancer mortality: a case-copntrol study. J Med Screening 5:99-103,1998.
53. Thompson IM, Zeidman EJ: Presentation and clinical course of patients ultimately succumbing to carcinoma of the prostate. Scand J Urol and Nephrol. 25:111-114,1991.
54. Jacobsen SJ, Katusic SK, Bergstralh EJ, et al: Incidence of prostate cancer diagnosis in the eras before and after serum prostate-specific antigen testing. J Am Med Assoc 274:1445-1449,1995.
55. Gann PH, Hennekens CH, Stampfer MJ, et al. A prospective evaluation of plasma PSA for detection of prostatic cancer. JAMA 273:289-294,1995.
56. Bartsch G, Horninger W, Klocker H, et al. Decrease in prostate cancer mortality following introduction of prostate specific antigen (PSA) screening in the federal state of Tyrol, Austria. Urology 58:417-424,2001.
57. Crawford ED, Leewansangtong S, Goktas S, et al.: Efficiency of prostate-specific antigen and digital rectal examination in screening, using 4.0 ng/ml and age-specific reference range as a cutoff for abnormal values. The Prostate 38(4): 296-302, 1999.
58. Schroder FH, van der Maas P, Beemsterboer P, et al.: Evaluation of the digital rectal examination as a screening test for prostate cancer. J Natl Cancer Inst 90:1817-1823,1998.
59. Breen N, Kessler L.: Changes in the use of screening mammography: evidence from 1987 and 1990 National Health Interview Surveys. Am J Pub Health 84:62-67,1994.
60. Barton MB, Harris R, Fletcher SW: Does this patient have breast cancer? The screening clinical breast cancer examination: should it be done,? How? JAMA 282:1270-1280,1999.
61. Thomas DB, Gao DL, Self SG, et al. Randomized trial of breast self-examination in Shanghai: methodology and preliminary results. JNCI 89:355-365,1997.
62. Newcomb PA, Weiss NS, Storer BE, et al. Breast self-examination in relation to the occurrence of advanced breast cancer. JNCI 83:260-265,1991.
63. Ellman R, Moss SM, Coleman D, et al. Breast self-examination programmes in the trial of early detection of breast cancer: ten year findings. British Journal of Cancer 1993; 68:208-12.
64. Miller AB, To T, Baines CJ , Wall C. Canadian National Breast Screening Study-2:13-Year results of randomized trial in Women aged 50-59 years. JNCI 92(18):1490-1499, 2000.
65. Rosenberg RD, Hunt WC, Williamson MR, et al. Effects of age, breast density, ethnicity, and estrogen replacement therapy on screening mammographic sensitivity and cancer stage at diagnosis: review of 183,134 screening mammograms in Albuquerque, New Mexico. Radiology 209:511-518,1998.

66. Hakama M, Holli K, Isola J, et al.: Aggressiveness of screen-detected breast cancers Lancet 345:221-224,1995.
67. Kerlikowske K, Grady D, Barclay J, et al. Likelihood ratios for modern screening mammography. Risk of breast cancer based on age and mammographic interpretation. JAMA 276:39-43,1996.
68. Kerlikowske K, Grady D, Barclay J, et al. Variability and accuracy in mammographic interpretation using the American College of Radiology Breast Imaging Reporting and Data System. JNCI 90:1801-1809,1998.
69. Elmore JG, Wells CK, Lee CH, et al. Variability in radiologists' interpretations of mammograms. NEJM 331:1493-1499,1994.
70. Elmore JG, Wells CK, Howard DH, et al. The impact of clinical history on mammographic interpretations. JAMA 277:49-52,1997.
71. Kerlikowske K, Grady D, Barclay J et al. Positive predictive value of screening mammography by age and family history of breast cancer. JAMA 270:2444-2450,1993.
72. Elmore JG, Barton MB, Moceri VM, et al. Ten-year risk of false positive screening mammograms and clinical breast examinations. NEJM 338:1089-1096,1998.
73. Welch HG, Fisher ES: Diagnostic testing following screening mammography in the elderly. JNCI 90:1389-1392,1998.
74. Pisano ED, Earp JA, Schell M, et al. Screening behavior of women after a false-positive mammogram. Radiol 208:245-249,1998.
75. Gotzsche PC, Olsen O: Is screening for breast cancer with mammography justifiable? Lancet 355:129-134,2000.
76. Statement of Andrew von Eschenbach, Director, National Cancer Institute before US Congress, February 28, 2002.
77. Tabar L, Vitak B, Chen HH, et al. Beyond randomized controlled trials: organized mammographic screening substantially reduces breast carcinoma mortality. Cancer 91:1699-703,2001.
78. Duffy SW. Tabar L, Chen HH, et al. The impact of organized mammography service screening on breast carcinoma mortality in seven Swedish counties. Cancer 95:458-469,2002.
79. Smith RA et al. American Cancer Society guidelines for the early detection of cancer. CA Cancer J Clin 52:8-22,2002.
80. http://cra.nci.nih.gov/6_printer/5_future_plans.htm.
81. Initiatives for molecular target drug discovery for cancer, http://grants1.nih.gov/grants/guide/pa-files/PAR-00-060.html
82. Blower PE, Yang C, Fligner MA, et al. Pharmacogenomic analysis: correlating molecular substructure classes with microarray gene expression data. Pharmacogenomics J 2002;2(4):259-71
83. Nowell PC, Hungerford DA: A minute chromosome in human chronic granulocytic leukemia. Science 132:1497-1501,1960.
84. Heisterkamp N, Jenster G, ten Hoeve, J. Acute leukemia in bcr/abl transgenic mice. Nature 344:251-253,1990.
85. Daley CQ, Van Etten RA, Baltimore D: Induction of chronic myelogenous leukemia in mice by the p210 bcr/abl gene of the Philadelphia chromosome, Science 247:824-830,1990.
86. Druker BJ, Talpaz M, Resta DJ, et al. Efficacy and safety of a specific inhibitor of the bcr/abl tyrosine kinase in chronic myeloid leukemia. N Engl J Med 344:1031-1037,2001.

87. O'Brien SG, Guilhot F, Larson RA, et al. Imatinib compared with interferon and low-dose cytarabine for newly diagnosed chronic-phase myeloid leukemia. N Engl J Med 348:1048-1050,2002.

88. Druker BJ, Talpaz, M, Resta DJ, et al. SRI571 (Gleevec ™) as a paradigm for cancer therapy. Trends in Mol Med 8(suppl):14-18,2002.

89. von bubnoff N, Schneller F, Peschel C, et al. Bcr-abl gene mutations in relation to clinical resistance of Philadelphia-chromosome-positive leukemia to STI571: a prospective study. The Lancet 359:487-491,2002.

90. Gorre ME, Mohammed M, Ellwood K, et al. Clinical resistance to STI571 cancer therapy caused by BCR-ABL gene mutation and amplification. Science 293:876-880,2001.

91. Hofman WK, de Vos S, Elashoff D, et al. Relation between resistance of Philadelphia-positive acute lymphoblastic leukaemia to the tyrosine kinase inibitor STI571 and gene-expression profiles: a gene-expression study. The Lancet 359:481-486,2002.

92. Hochhaus A, Cony-Makhoul P, Melo JV, et al. Roots of clinical resistance to STI-571 cancer therapy. Science 293:2163,2001.

93. Mauro MJ et al. STI571: A paradigm of new agents for cancer therapeutics. J Clin Oncol 20: 325-334,2002.

94. Heinrich MC, Blanke CD, Druker BJ, et al. Inhibition of KIT tyrosine kinase activity: a novel molecular approach to the treatment of KIT-positive malignancies. J Clin Oncol 20:1692-703,2002

95. Blanke CD, von Mehren M, Joensuu H, et al. Evaluation of the safety and efficacy of an oral molecularly-targeted therapy (STI571), in patients with unresectable or metastatic gastrointestinal stromal tumors (GISTS) expressing c-KIT (CD117). Proc Am Soc Clin Onc 20:1a, 2001.

96. International Human Genome Sequencing Consortium. Initial sequencing and analysis of the human genome. Nature 409:860-921,2001.

97. Venter JC, Adams MD, Meyers EW, et al. The sequence of the human genome, Science 291:1304-1351, 2001.

98. Drews J. Drug discovery: A historical perspective. Science 287:1960-1964,2000.

99. Bailey D, Zanders E, Dean P. The end of the beginning for genomic medicine. Nat Biotechnol 19:207-209,2001.

100. Foster BA, Coffey HA, Morin MJ, et al. Pharmacological rescue of mutant p53 conformation and function. Science 286:2507-2510,1999.

101. Khuri FR, Nemunaitis J, Ganly I, et al. A controlled trial of intratumoral Onyx-015, a selective-replication adenovirus, in combination with cisplatin and 6-fluorouracil in patients with recurrent head and neck cancer. Nat Med 6:879-885,2000.

102. Harries M, Smith I. The development and clinical use of trastuzumab (Herceptin). Endocr Relat Cancer. 2002 Jun;9(2):75-85

103. Slamon D, Leyland-Jones B, Shak S, et al. Use of chemotherapy plus a monoclonal antibody against HER2 for metastatic breast cancer that over-expresses HER2. New Engl J Med 344:783-792,2001.

104. Ewer MS, Gibbs HR, Swafford J, et al. Cardiotoxicity of patients receiving transtumumab (Herceptin): primary toxicity, synergism, sequential stress, or surveillance artifact? Semin Oncol 26:96-101,1999.
105. Gibbs JB Mechanism-based target identification and drug discovery in cancer research. Science 287:1969-1973,2000.
106. Workman P. Scoring the bull's-eye against cancer genome targets. Curr Opin Pharmacol 1:342-352,2001.
107. Kipps TJ. Gene therapy in Chronic Lymphocytic Leukemia: Advances in Genetics, Biology, and Management, Ed GB Faguet, Humana Press, 2003.
108. Alizadeh AA, Eisen MB, Davis RE, et al. Distinct types of diffuse B-cell lymphoma identified by gene expression profiling. Nature (Lond.) 403:503-511,2000.
109. Hamblin, T.J., Davis, Z., Gardiner, A., et al. Unmutated Ig V(H) genes are associated with a more aggressive form of chronic lymphocytic leukemia. Blood 1999; 94:1848-1854.
110. Connors T. Anticancer drugs development: The way forward. The Oncologist 1:180-181,1996.
111. Chen GQ, Shi XG, Tang W, et al. Use of arsenic trioxide (As203) in the treatment of acute promyelocytic leukemia (APL). I. As203 exerts dose-dependent dual effects of APL cells. Blood 89:3345-3353,1997.
112. Adjei AA, Davis JN, Erlishman C, et al. Farnesyl transferase inhibition: use of surrogate markers. Proc Am Soc Cancer Res Plenary 9, 1999.
113. Adjei AA, Erlishman C, Davis JN, et al. A phase I trial of farnesyl transferase inhibitor SCH66336: evidence for biological and clinical activity. Cancer Res 60:1871-1877,2000.
114. Spiro TP, Gerson SL, Liu L, et al. O^6-benxylguanine: A clinical trial establishing the biochemical modulatory dose in tumor tissue for alkyltransferase-directed DNA repair. Cancer Res 59:2402-2410,1999.
115. Simon R. Optimal two-stage designs for phase II clinical trials. Control Clin Trials 10:1-10,1989.
116. Baidas SM, Winer EP, Fleming GF, et al. Phase II evaluation of thalidomide in patients with metastatic breast cancer. J Clin Oncol 18:2710-2717,2000.
117. Simon R. New method for the design and analysis of clinical trials. Principles Practice Oncol Updates 13:1-9,1999.
118. Kopec JA, Abrahamwicz M, Esdaile JM. Randomized discontinuation trials: Utility and efficiency. J Clin Epidemiol 46:959-971,1993.
119. Improving Palliative Care for Cancer. Foley KM, Gelband H, editors. National Cancer Policy board - National Research Council, National Academic Press, Washington, D.C., 2001.
120. Singer PA, Martin DK, Kelner M. Quality end-of-life care: patients' perspectives. JAMA 281:163-8,1999.
121. Teno JM, Fisher ES, Hamel MB, et al. Medical care inconsistent with patients' treatment goals: Association with 1-year Medicare resource use and survival. J Am Ger Soc 50:496-500,2002.
122. Walsh D, Donnelly S, Rybicki L. The symptoms of advanced cancer: Relationship to age, gender, and performance status in 1,000 patients. Support Care Cancer 8:175-179,2000.

123. Portenoy RK, Thaler HT, Kornblitch AB, et al. Symptom prevalence, characteristics and distress in a cancer population. Qual Life Res 3:183-190,1994.
124. WHO definition of palliative care, http://www.who.int/dsa/justpub/cpl.htm
125. Burnett A, Büchner T. Risk adapted treatment of acute myeloid leukemia. Program. 7th Congress of the European Haematology Association; June 6-9,2002; Florence, Italy.
126. Dighiero G. Clinical management: Guidelines in Chronic Lymphocytic Leukemia: Advances in Molecular genetics, Biology, Diagnosis, and Management. Ed Guy B Faguet, Humana Press, Totowa, NJ, 2003.

GLOSSARY

Reproduced with permission and adaptations, from: DOE Human Genome Program – www.ornl.gov/hgmi), ACS (www.cancer.org), and other public domain sources.

A

Adenine (A): A nitrogenous base, one member of the base pair AT (adenine-thymine).

Adenocarcinoma: Cancer that arises from glandular tissue, such as in the ducts or lobules of the breast or the lining cells of the intestine.

Adjuvant therapy: Treatment that is added to the primary treatment to increase effectiveness (e.g. chemotherapy to enhance radiation therapy, or vice versa).

Advanced cancer: Refers to cancer that has spread locally or to distant parts of the body. The latter is also called metastatic cancer.

Allele: One of two DNA sequences inherited separately from each parent that together are responsible for a particular inherited trait. Alleles can be normal (most common, such as eye color) or mutated (very rare, as in retinoblastoma).

Amino acid: Any of a class of 20 molecules that are combined to form proteins in living things. The sequence of amino acids in a protein and hence protein function are determined by the *genetic code*.

Amplification: An increase in the number of copies of a specific DNA fragment.

Angiogenesis: New blood vessel formation that promotes cancer growth.

Antibody or immunoglobulin: A protein produced by B-Lymphocytes in response to antigens found on the surface of foreign agents, such as bacteria or mismatched transplanted tissues. See *Lymphocytes*.

Antigen: A substance that causes the body's immune system to react by producing antibodies. See *Lymphocytes, T-Lymphocytes, B- Lymphocytes*.

Apoptosis or programmed cell death: A normal, genetically controlled process that causes a cell to die when its DNA is damaged.

Autosome: One of 22 pairs of chromosomes not involved in sex determination.

Autosomal dominant (gene): A gene on a non-sex chromosome that is always expressed if passed to an offspring. It is responsible for inherited dominant traits or illnesses, if mutated (the carrier is said to be heterozygous for the trait or mutation). It is inherited by 1 out of 2 offsprings.

Autosomal recessive (inheritance): A non-dominant gene that requires both copies (one inherited from each parent) in order to express a trait or illness, if mutated (the carrier is said to be homozygous for the trait or mutation). It is inherited by 1 out of 4 offsprings.

B

B-Lymhocytes: One of two major types of lymphocytes. See *Lymphocytes, T-Lymphocytes.*

Base pair (bp): Two nitrogenous bases (AT or GC) held together by weak bonds. The two DNA strands are held together in the shape of a double helix by the bonds between base pairs.

Benign tumor: A non-cancerous tissue growth that does not spread distally.

Biologic response modifiers: Agents that enhance the immune system to fight cancer. **Biotechnology:** A set of biological techniques developed for research and product development, such as recombinant DNA, cell fusion, and bioprocessing techniques.

Bone marrow transplant: Infusion of bone marrow cells to enable high-dose cancer chemotherapy that also destroys the patient's bone marrow. The transplant is called *allogeneic* when cells originate from a matched donor; *autologous* when they are the patient's own, and *syngeneic* when they derive from an identical twin.

C

Cancer: A group of over 200 diseases caused by mutations of critical genes that confer a growth or survival advantage to the affected cells. See *Neoplasm, Tumor*.

Carcinogens: Agents, regardless of type and nature, that cause cancer. The most lethal chemical carcinogen worldwide is tobacco.

Carcinoma in situ: Cancer in its earliest recognizable stage that, given its confinement to the cells where it began with no spread to surrounding tissues, is highly curable. See *In situ*.

Chemotherapy: Treatment with drugs aimed at destroy cancer cells. Most chemotherapy drugs inhibit cell proliferation through disruption of the cell-cycle.

Chromosomes: Self-replicating microscopic structures bundled in the cell nucleus that consist of genes. In humans, 23 pairs of chromosomes, each pair containing one chromosome inherited from each parent, carry the entire genetic code.

Clone: An exact copy made of biological material such as a DNA segment , a whole cell, or a complete organism. See *Monoclonal.*

Cloning: A specialized DNA technology that enables production of exact copies of a single gene (clone libraries), a cell (cell lines), or an entire organism (Dolly the sheep).

Codon: See Genetic code.

Computed-assisted tomography (CAT or CT scan). A non-invasive imaging technique that uses x-rays to produce two-dimensional images of internal organs or structures.

Cure: To heal or restored to health. From an Oncology standpoint, cure is equated to continuous disease-free survival lasting 5 years or longer after completion of treatment.

Cytosine (C): A nitrogenous base that is a member of the base pair GC (guanine and cytosine).

Cytokines: Cell-secreted proteins that act as intracellular mediator signals.

D

Diploid: A full set of genetic material, consisting of paired chromosomes, one from each parent. The diploid human genome has 46 chromosomes or twice the haploid. See *Haploid.*

DNA (deoxyribonucleic acid): DNA is a double stranded molecule, held together by weak bonds between base pairs of nucleotides (AT and GC), that encodes genetic information.

DNA probe: Single-stranded DNA or RNA molecules of specific base sequence, labeled either radioactively or immunologically, that are used to detect the complementary base sequence by hybridization.

DNA sequence: The relative order of base pairs, whether in a fragment of DNA, a gene, a chromosome, or an entire genome.

Double helix: The shape that two linear strands of DNA assume when bonded together.

E

Embryonal tumors: Tumors that exhibit tissues present in the developing fetus and occur mostly in children or young adults.

Endonuclease: An enzyme that cleaves its nucleic acid substrate at internal sites in the nucleotide sequence.

Enzyme: A protein that acts as a catalyst, speeding the rate of a biochemical reaction without altering its nature or direction.

Eukaryote: Cell or organism with membrane bound, structurally discrete nucleus and other well-developed subcellular compartments. Eukaryotes include all organisms except viruses, bacteria, and blue-green algae. See Prokaryote.

Exon: The protein coding DNA sequence of a gene. See Intron.

Exonuclease: An enzyme that cleaves nucleotides sequentially from free ends of a linear nucleic acid substrate.

F

FISH (fluorescence in situ hybridization): Use of fluorescing RNA or DNA probes to detect complementary sequences. Its is valuable for chromosome mapping.

Flow cytometry: Analysis of biological material by detection of the light-absorbing or fluorescing properties of cells or subcellular fractions (i.e., chromosomes) passing in a narrow stream through a laser beam. Cell type and origin can be ascertained based on their absorbance or fluorescence profiles.

Fusion (or chimeric) gene: A gene made of several parts not normally found together. It is usually the result of gene translocation associated with malignancies.

G

Gamete: Mature male or female reproductive cell (sperm or ovum) with a haploid set of chromosomes (23 for humans). See Gonads.

Gene: An ordered nucleotide sequence on the DNA molecule that encodes a specific functional product (i.e., a protein or RNA molecule). Genes are the physical and functional unit of heredity passed from parent to offspring.

Gene expression: The process by which a gene's coded information is transcribed into mRNA, whether or not the transcription is translated into protein synthesis.

Gene family: Group of closely related genes that make similar products.

Gene product: The biochemical material, either RNA or protein, that results from expression of a gene.

Gene therapy: An experimental procedure aimed at replacing, manipulating, or supplementing defective genes with healthy ones.

Genetic code: The sequence of nucleotides, coded in triplets (cordons) along the mRNA, that determines the sequence of amino acids in protein synthesis.

Genetics: The study of the mechanisms of heredity and biological variation.

Genome: All the genetic material, housed in the chromosomes, of a particular organism.

Genomic sequence: The order of the subunits, called bases, that makes up a particular fragment of DNA in a genome. The particular sequence of bases encodes important information in an individual's genetic blueprint, and is unique for each individual (except identical twins).

Germ cell: See Gamete.

Gonads: Sex organs (ovary and testicle), which produces the gametes in most multicellular animals. See gametes.

Guanine (G): A nitrogenous base, one member of the base pair GC (guanine and cytosine).

H

Haploid: A single set of chromosomes (half the full set of genetic material), present in the egg and sperm cells of animals and in the egg and pollen cells of plants. Human's reproductive cells have 23 chromosomes. Compare *Diploid*.

Heterozygosity: Having two different alleles of the same gene. See *Allele*. See *Gene*.

Heterozygote: An individual expressing heterozygosity. Heterozygotes can have one normal and one mutated allele, or a different mutation on each allele (double heterozygote).

Hodgkin's disease: A cancer characterized by progressive, sequential, and painless enlargement of lymph nodes, spleen, and liver. See *Non-Hodgkin's lymphoma*

Homology: Similarity in DNA or protein sequences between individuals of the same species or among different species.

Homologous chromosome: Chromosome containing the same linear gene sequences as another, each derived from one parent.

Homozygote: An individual that has two identical alleles of a gene. See *Heterozygoye*.

Homozygous genotype: Occurs when both alleles at a particular gene locus are the same. A person may be homozygous for the normal allele or for a mutation.

Human Genome Project: A multinational research and technology development effort, coordinated by the National Institutes of Health and the Department of Energy, aimed at mapping and sequencing some or all of the genome of human beings and other organisms.

Hybridization: The process of joining two complementary strands of DNA or one each of DNA and RNA to form a double-stranded molecule. See *Southern blotting*.

I

Immune enhancers: See *Biological response modifiers.*

Immune system: The highly complex network of specialized cells and organs that defend the body against attacks by "foreign" invaders such as bacteria, viruses, and transplanted tissues. See *Antibody* and *Antigen.*

Immunotherapy: A medical technique aimed at stimulating the immune system to attack and destroy disease-causing cells (including viruses, bacteria, and cancer cells)

Informatics: The application of computer and statistical techniques to the management of information. In genome projects, informatics includes the development of methods to quickly search databases, analyze DNA sequence information, and to predict protein sequence and structure from DNA sequence data.

In situ: From Latin *in place.* See *Carcinoma in situ* and *In situ hybridization.*

In situ hybridization: See *Fluorescence In situ hybridization.*

Incidence: The number of new cases of a disease that occurs among a population during a certain period of time.

Interphase: The period in the cell cycle when DNA is replicated in the nucleus. It includes all phases of the cell-cycle but mitosis. See *metaphase.*

Intron: The DNA sequence in a eukaryotic gene that is not translated into a protein. See *Exon.*

In vitro: Outside a living organism.

K

Karyotype: A photomicrograph of an individual's chromosomes arranged in a standard format showing the number, size, and shape of each chromosome type. It is used to identify gross chromosomal abnormalities known to occur in specific diseases.

Kilobase (kb): Unit of length for DNA fragments equal to 1,000 nucleotides.

L

Locus: The position a gene, DNA, or other marker on a chromosome. See *Gene expression.*

Lymphatic system: A system of vessels, organs (including, lymph nodes, spleen, thymus, and bone marrow), that produce, store, and carry mainly lymphocytes. Cancer cells can spread through lymphatic channels, invading first lymph nodes and later distant organs.

Lymphocytes: A type of white blood cells that originate in the lymphatic system and are at the core of immune reactions. There are two major types of lymphocytes: B-cells that produce antibodies, and T-cells that are mainly responsible for foreign tissue rejection. See B-*Lymphocytes, T-Lymphocytes*.

Lymphokines: A class of cytokines secreted by T-cells in response to antigen stimulation that act as intercellular signals of the immune system. See *Cytokines, T-cells*.

Lymphoma: A group of cancers arising from the lymphatic system. There are two main types: Hodgkin's disease and Non-Hodgkin's lymphoma. The former is mostly curable. The latter, which affects mostly B-lymphocytes, includes more than 20 different variants ranging from indolent forms compatible with a multi-year survival, to rapidly fatal aggressive forms. See *Hodgkin's disease, Non-Hodgkin's lymphoma*.

M

Magnetic resonance imaging: A non-invasive imaging technique that uses radio waves to produce two-dimensional images of internal organs or structures. See *CT scans*.

Mammogram or mammography: A diagnostic procedure for detecting X-ray evidence of breast tumors. Its main application is for *Screening* for the presence of non-palpable tumors.

Marker: An identifiable physical location on a chromosome (e.g., restriction enzyme cutting site, gene) whose inheritance can be monitored.

Meiosis: The form of cell division occurring in sex cells that leads to the production of gametes. See *Mitosis, Gametes*.

Medical Oncology: The subspecialty within Internal Medicine that studies and treats cancer.

Messenger RNA (mRNA): The class of RNA that copies the genetic code from nuclear DNA and serves as a template for protein synthesis in cytoplasmic ribosomes. See *RNA, DNA*.

Metaphase: A stage in mitosis or meiosis during which the chromosomes are aligned along the equatorial plane of the cell. See *Mitosis, Meiosis*.

Metastasis The spread of cancer from its original site to distant sites via lymphatic or blood vessels.

Microarrays: Also referred to as Biochip, DNA chip, DNA microarray, and Gene or Genome array, are microplatforms that use probes with known targets to test DNA fragments, antibodies, or proteins. Their applications include gene discovery and profiling, disease diagnosis, pharmacogenomics, and toxicogenomics.

Mitosis: The process of nuclear division that produces daughter cells that is genetically identical to each other and to the parent cell. See *meiosis*.

Monoclonal: Derived from a single clone. See *Clone*.

Myeloid, myelocytic, or myelogenous leukemias: A group of chronic or acute leukemias affecting myeloid cells, a type of blood cells originating in the bone marrow.

Mutation: An alteration in DNA structure or sequence of a gene. Mutations can be beneficial, neutral, or harmful, and can be inherited if they occur in eggs or sperm. Certain mutations may lead to cancer or other diseases.

N

Neoplasm or Neoplasia: Any new and abnormal tissue growth. These terms and cancer are used interchangeably. See *tumor*.

Nitrogenous base: A nitrogen-containing molecule having the chemical properties of a base.

Non-Hodgkin's lymphoma: See *Lymphoma, Hodgkin's disease*.

Nucleic acid: A large molecule composed of nucleotide subunits. See Nucleotide.

Nucleotide: A subunit of DNA or RNA consisting of a nitrogenous base (adenine, guanine, thymine, or cytosine in DNA (adenine, guanine, uracil, or cytosine in RNA), a phosphate molecule, and a sugar molecule (deoxyribose in DNA and ribose in RNA). Thousands of nucleotides are linked to form a DNA or RNA molecule. See *DNA, Base-pair, RNA*.

Nucleus: The cellular organelle in eukaryotes that contains the all chromosomes and their genetic material.

O

Oncogene: A mutated proto-oncogene that contributes to cancer formation. See *Proto-Oncogene, Tumor suppressor gene*.

P

Palliation: Alleviation of symptoms caused by the disease or its treatment.

Penetrance: The probability of a gene or genetic trait being expressed.

Permucosal: Performed through mucosa, as dental anesthesia.

Percutaneous: Performed through the skin, as an injection or a biopsy.

Pharmacogenomics: The study of the interaction of an individual's genetic makeup and response to a drug. The ultimate goal of pharmacogenomics research is to help tailor medicines to a person's unique genetic make-up.

Placebo: A medically inert substance given for psychological benefit or as part of a clinical research study. Perceived improvement while taking placebos is referred to as *placebo effect*.

Polymerase chain reaction (PCR): A method that enzymatically amplifies a DNA base sequence. Through amplification PCR enables detection of minute amounts of DNA sequences not otherwise detectable. See *Polymerase*.

Polymerase (DNA or RNA): An enzymes that catalyze the synthesis of nucleic acids on preexisting nucleic acid templates, assembling RNA from ribonucleotides or DNA from deoxyribonucleotides.

Polymorphism: A difference in DNA sequence (or "common" mutation) with a frequency of at least 1% in the population. See *Mutation*.

Positron emission tomography (PET): A computerized imaging technique that depicts the metabolic activity in various tissues. See *CT-scan, MRI*.

Prevalence: The total number of people in a population with a given disease at a given time.

Probe: Single-stranded DNA or RNA sequences, labeled radioactively or immunologically that are used to detect the presence of complementary nucleotide sequences. See *Nucleotide*.

Prokaryote: A cell, more primitive than a eukaryote, having no nucleus. Prokaryotes include bacteria and blue-green algae. See *Eukaryote*.

Prognosis: A prediction of the course of a disease. *Prognostic indicators* such as disease stage and patient age cab be valuable tools for planning disease management.

Prostate specific antigen (PSA): A protein made by the prostate gland. Because PSA blood levels may be elevated in prostate cancer, it is a useful screening tool.

Protein: A large molecule composed of amino acids in a specific sequence. Proteins are required for the structure, function, and regulation of cells, tissues, and organs. Examples include hormones, enzymes, and antibodies. See *amino acid*.

Proteome: The full complement of proteins produced by a particular genome.

Proto-Oncogene: A gene that usually codes for a regulatory protein. It becomes an oncogene if it mutates. See *Oncogene, Tumor suppressor genes*.

Purine: A nitrogen-containing, double-ring, basic compound that occurs in nucleic acids. The purines in DNA and RNA are adenine and guanine. See *Pyrimidine*.

Pyrimidine: A nitrogen-containing, single-ring, basic compound that occurs in nucleic acids. The pyrimidines in DNA are cytosine and thymine; in RNA, cytosine and uracil. See *Purine*.

R

Recombinant: *Recombinant clone*, Clone containing recombinant DNA molecules. *Recombinant DNA,* The process of cutting and recombining DNA fragments from different sources as a means to isolate genes or to alter their structure and function, or transfer genetic material from on organism to another. *Recombinant DNA technology:* Procedure used to join together DNA segments in a cell-free system. See *Clone, DNA*.

Remission: A period or state during which detectable disease and symptoms decrease (partial remission) of subside (complete remission).

Retina: Light-sensitive layer of tissue located at the back of the eye that transmits visual images to the brain.

Ribonucleic acid (RNA): A large DNA-like molecule found in the nucleus and cytoplasm of cells. Several classes of RNA molecules, including *messenger RNA, transfer RNA, ribosomal RNA*, and other small RNAs, play an important role in protein synthesis and other activities of the cell. See *DNA, Ribosomes.*

Ribosome: Cellular organelle that is the site of protein synthesis during mRNA translation.
See *mRNA, Translation.*

S

Sequencing: Determination of the order of nucleotides (base sequences) in a DNA or RNA molecule or the order of amino acids in a protein. See *DNA, RNA, Nucleotides.*

Sex chromosomes: The two chromosomes that determine sex (XX in women and XY in men).

Somatic cell: Any cell in the body except gametes and their precursors. See *Gamete*

Southern blotting: A procedure in which DNA fragments are transferred from an agarose gel to a nitrocellulose filter, where the denatured DNA is then hybridized to a radioactive probe (blotting). See *Hybridization.*

Sporadic cancer: Cancer that occurs randomly and is not inherited from parents.

Stage: The measurement of the extent of a cancer. It ranges from in situ to disseminated or metastatic cancer. See *Carcinoma in situ, Metastasis.*

T

T-Lymphocyes: One of two major types of lymphocytes. See *Lymphocytes, B-Lymphocytes.*

Telomere: A specialized stretch of repeated DNA sequences at the end of a chromosome that shortens with each cell division, controlling the cell life-span.

Telomerase: An enzyme that restores and maintains telomere length in some undifferentiated cells such as embryonic and stem cells and in cancer cells.

Thymine (T): A nitrogenous base, one member of the base pair AT (adenine-thymine).

Transcription: The synthesis of an RNA copy from a sequence of DNA (a gene); the first step in gene expression. See *Translation.*

Transformation: A process by which the genetic material carried by an individual cell is altered by incorporation of exogenous DNA into its genome. The term is also applied clinically to the evolution of cancer from a relatively indolent form to an aggressive one.

Translation: The process in which the genetic code carried by mRNA directs the synthesis of proteins from amino acids in the cytoplasmic ribosome. See *Ribosome, Transcription.*

Tumor: An abnormal tissue growth that can be benign or malignant. See *Neoplasm, Cancer.*

Tumor suppressor genes: Genes that normally balance the effects of growth-promoting proteins. When absent or dysfunctional, they can contribute to cancer development. See *Proto-Oncogenes, Oncogenes.*

V

Virus: A piece of DNA or RNA wrapped in a thin protein coat that invades living cells and uses cellular mechanisms to create multiple copies of itself. Retroviruses are RNA viruses that utilize the enzyme reverse transcriptase to reverse-copy its genome into a DNA intermediate, which integrates into the host cell chromosome. Many naturally occurring cancers are caused by retroviruses.

INDEX

Printed in the United States
65777LVS00002B/211-234